8-9-96

Dear Alice,

Best Wishes to you and you

[illegible signature]

AF694690

Beyond The Dark Cloud

Road To Recovery From
Chronic Fatigue and Immune Dysfunction
After 25 Years

By Thea Schlosser

Foreword by internationally acclaimed pioneer and researcher on Chronic Fatigue and Immune Dysfunction and founder of the Chronic Fatigue Institute
Jay Goldstein, M.D.

Preface by recognized pioneer of the impact of negative and positive emotions on the immune system and the need for healing
Lona Peoples

Introduction by world-famed scientist, researcher and expert on Neuro-Immunology and pioneer on Xenotransplant Therapy
Professor Wolfram Kühnau, M.D.

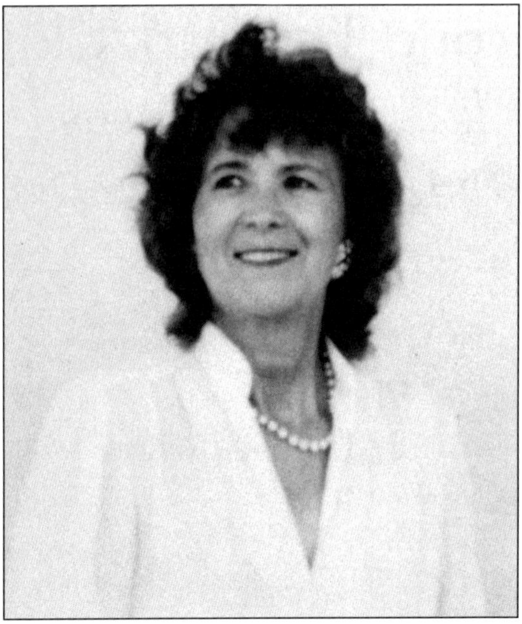

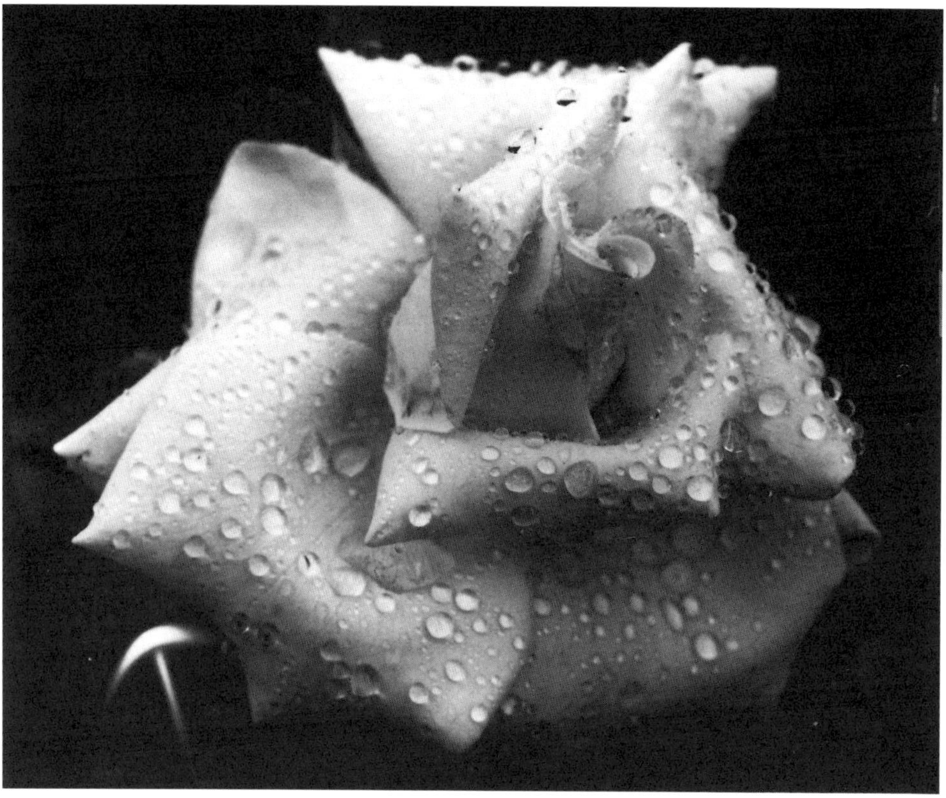

Photo by Thea. "The Inspiration of a Rose." (Black and White)

Cover photograph by Thea Schlosser
Book cover by Angie Burke-Graphic Design
Book production by Evelyn Bradley, Graphic Traffic
Printing by Haagen Printing

Chronic Fatigue and Immune Dysfunction
Media Awareness Association Press
P.O. Box 41028
Santa Barbara, California 93140

LOOK FOR US SOON ON THE INTERNET.

Phone or Fax (805) 963-7799 or Fax (805) 969-7669

© 1995 Chronic Fatigue and Immune Dysfunction Media Awareness Association Press. All rights reserved. This book is protected by copyright. No part of it may be reproduced or stored in any kind of computer or retrieval system, in any form or by any means, electronic, photocopied or otherwise, without the prior written permission of the publisher.

Printed in the United States of America
First Printing—May 1996

ISBN 0-9653215-0-9

A Note To The Reader

Please always undertake diet, exercise, or anything else suggested in this book with your licensed and qualified health care provider. What works for one person may not necessarily work well for another. This book should not be a substitute for professional advice and treatment. The author and publisher cannot accept legal responsibility for the above reason.

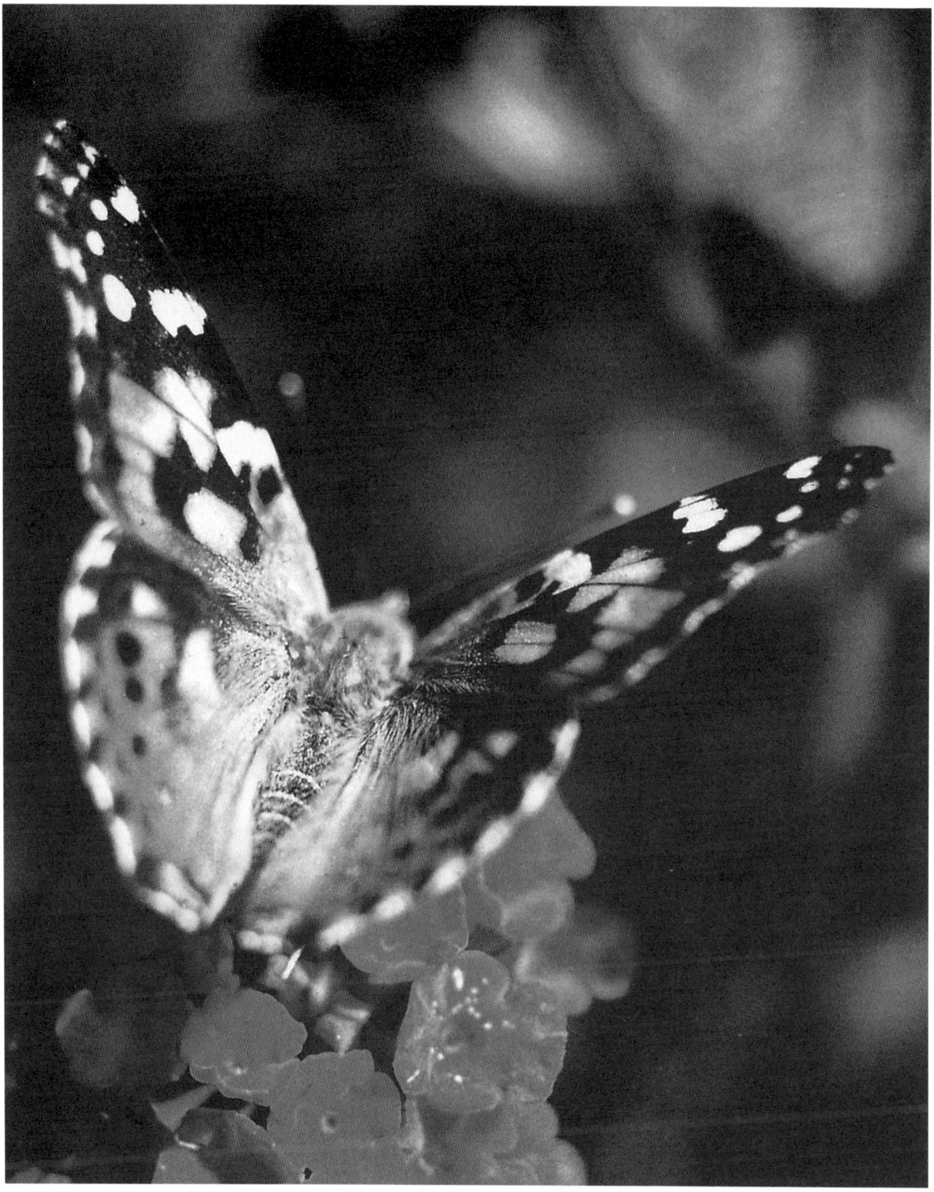

Photo by Thea.

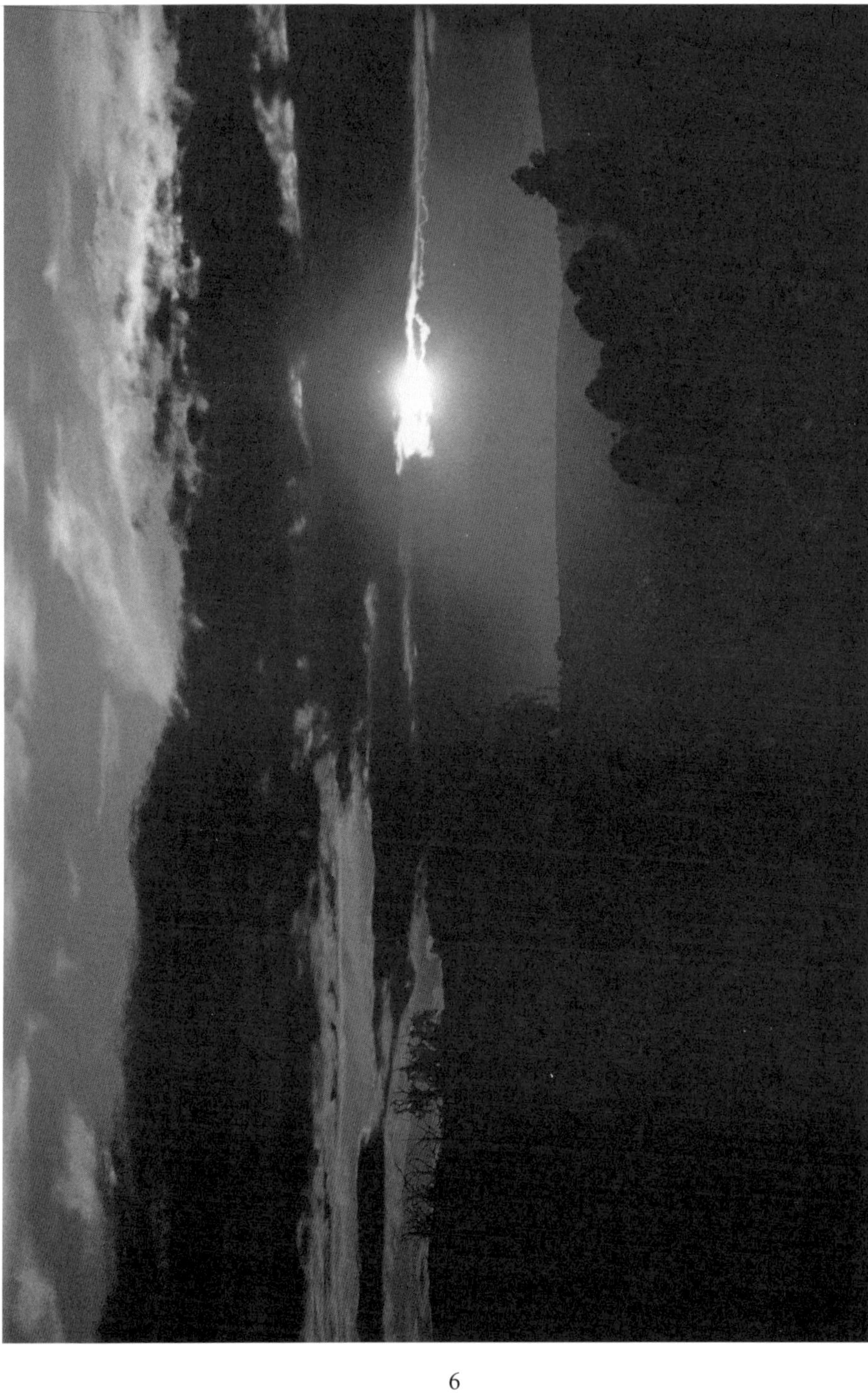

Cover Photo by Thea: Sunset in Santa Barbara, California.

Beyond The Dark Cloud

There is a gray cloud
Darkening my life
Cannot work, cannot sleep,
Cannot think anymore.
Enjoying my life was cut,
Like with a knife.
Desperately seeking a way out,
A door!

Everything is hurting—including my bones.
No doctor can help me escape
From the night.
I am so helpless, I am so alone.
But now I see, that I have to fight!

There are other people who suffer like me.
New knowledge, a storm will erase darkness and rain.
New medical thinking is coming I see
New hope that the sun
Will shine on me again.

Written for me by Professor Wolfram Kühnau, M.D., 1994

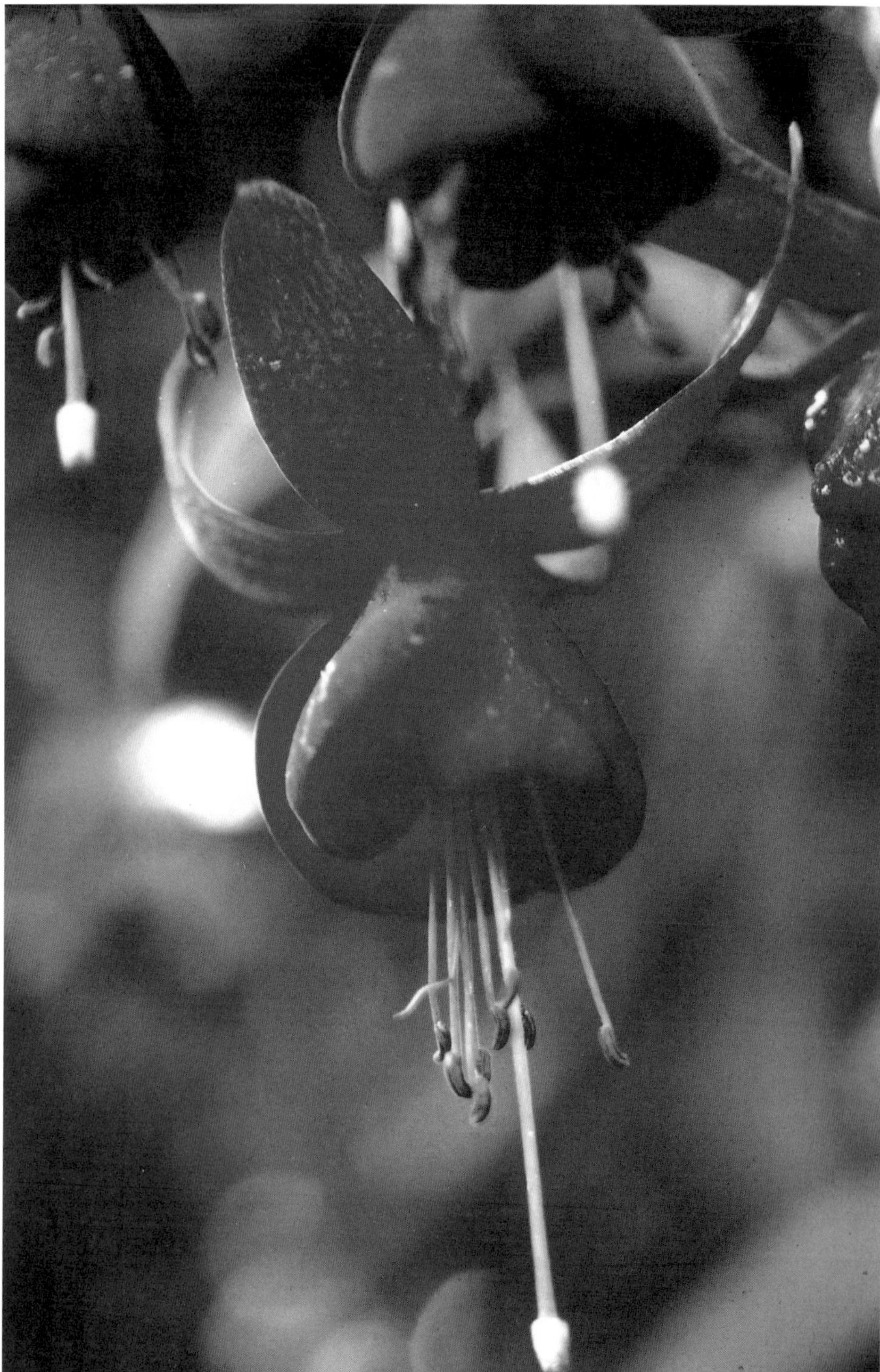

Photo by Thea.

"Beyond The Dark Cloud" is dedicated to:

❦

❦ My family—the center point of my life.

❦ Mama and Papa who endured, lost, and suffered so much to raise us children.

❦ My sisters, Anneliese and Maria.

❦ Hugo and Ida Hermesmeyer, my brother and sister-in-law.

❦ My mother-in-law and father-in-law, Karl and Katarina Schlosser.

❦ You, the Chronic Fatigue survivor, for your courage to overcome this illness.

❦ You, who do not have Chronic Fatigue, but support a loved one who does.

❦ Professor Wolfram Kühnau, M.D.

❦ The Medical Pioneers—who believed that Chronic Fatigue DOES exist—and never gave up on us.

❦ My friend Lona Peoples—for her love and support, her outstanding work with healing of old hurts, and her beautiful preface.

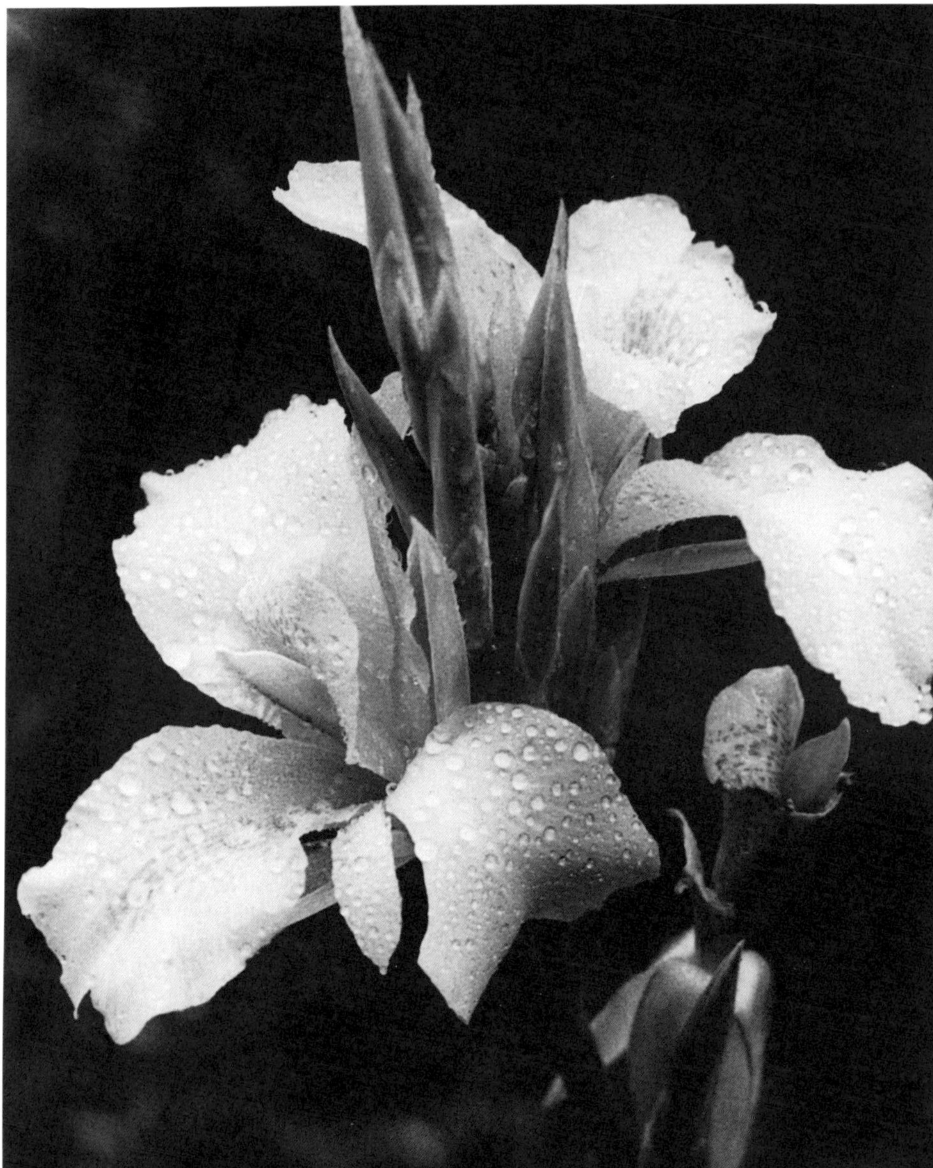

Photo by Thea. (Black and White)

ꕥ Erika Perkins, my dear friend,
for all her love and compassion.

ꕥ Sibylle Vilucci, my special friend, for her
encouragement, love, support, and compassion.

ꕥ Mr. Rich Carson, founder of the CFIDS Buyer's Club,
the largest fund-raiser for CFIDS.

ꕥ CFIDS Society of America: To my knowledge,
the largest organization committed to helping
CFIDS survivors.

ꕥ And last but not least: all of the wonderful health care
providers who are dedicated to finding an answer
and cure for CFIDS. I am sorry that I cannot
list all of you. I truly believe that had it
not been for the efforts and brilliance
of these people, many of us
could not have survived.

Thank You So Very Much.
Peace and Health To You.
God Bless You All.

—Thea

My Deepest Appreciation to:

❧ My caring, loving daughter Ingrid and her husband Steven Boehm for their enormous love and support. I can easily say that without their support I might not be here today.

❧ My loving daughter Evelyn, whom I call Elly, and her husband Mike, for all their love and support.

❧ Karl, my ex-husband, for his never-ending support.

❧ My loving grandchildren Shane, Chris, Jeff, and Ryan, who always fill my heart with joy.

❧ My sister Anneliese Narath, who never gave up encouraging me through her love and support, as well as her children Margaret, Karin, and Alex, and their families.

❧ My sister Maria Rechbauer, her husband Anton, her son Peter, and her daughter Carmen, Carmen's husband Gary and son Robert, from Australia, for their love and encouragement.

❧ Dr. and Mrs. Eric Boehm, for all of their love and encouragement.

- Wally and Jerry Prukop, for their love and support.

- So many of my friends, who took care of my dear children, especially Maria and Anton Bajhart, as well as Marian Dolce and her family, and Adam and Barbara Quintus.

Quite frankly, there are too many to name you all, but may I express a special thanks to all of you, and may God bless you always.

With my deepest thanks and gratitude–

Love and Peace,
Thea

A Special Thanks to the Following Contributors:

Jay Goldstein, M.D., for his loving foreword and his very helpful questionnaire on CFIDS.

Professor Wolfram Kühnau, M.D., for his heartwarming introduction, his lovely poem and for his articles on Double Blind Studies and Live-Cell Therapy and brain sketch. Over the years, he has been a tremendous support and friend.

Henry Hoegerman, M.D., "Chronic Fatigue and the Candida Connection."

Dr. Nephtali Solis, "Homeopathy: A Natural Medicine."

Roy Kupsinel, M.D., "Mercury—Amalgam Toxicity."

Steve Boehm, President of Efficient Systems, "The Importance of Proper Nutrition."

Bari Maddock, "This I Know."

Lucy Campa, "Aromatherapy."

Arlen L. Bass, D.O., "Osteopathy."

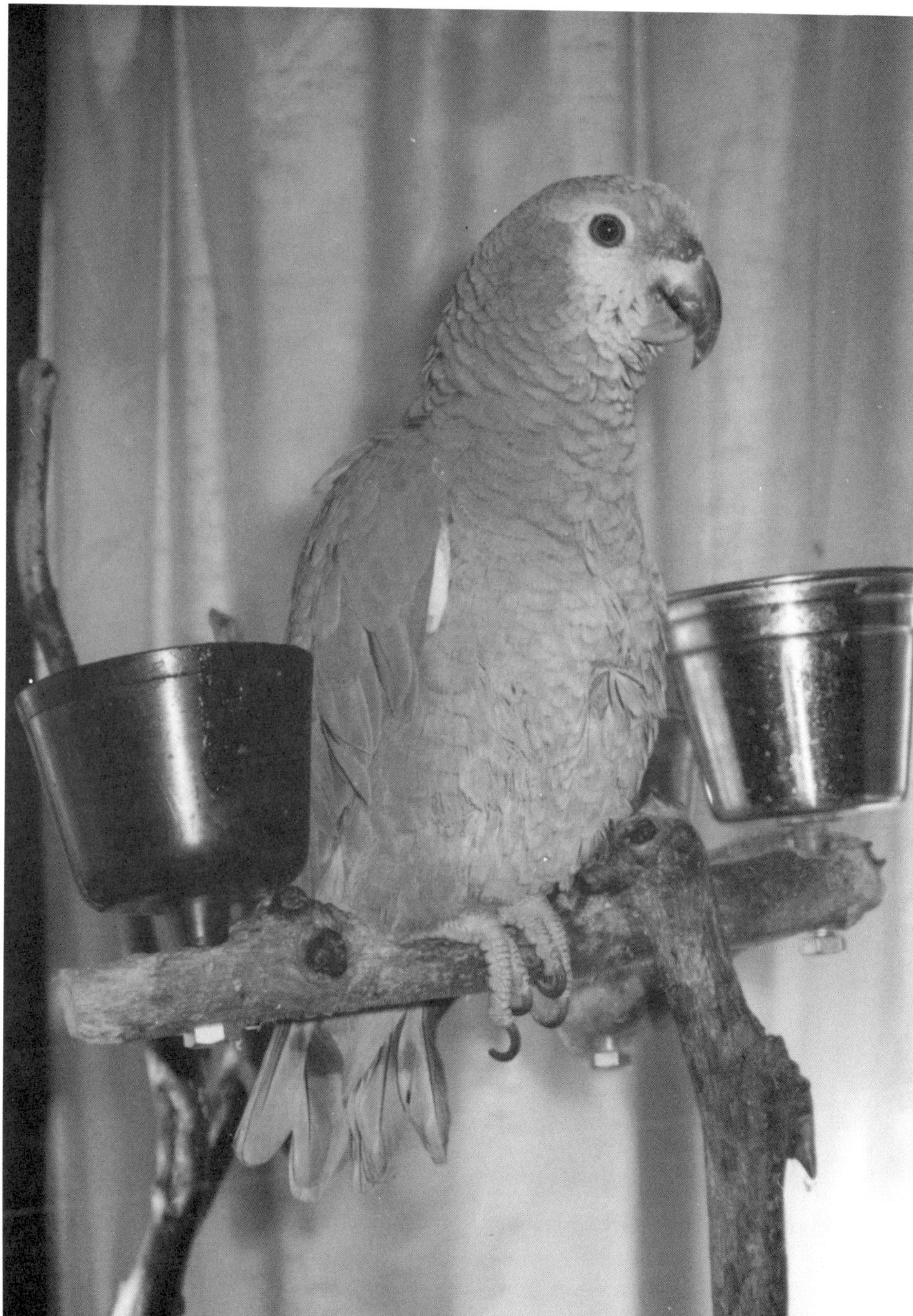

Photo by Thea.

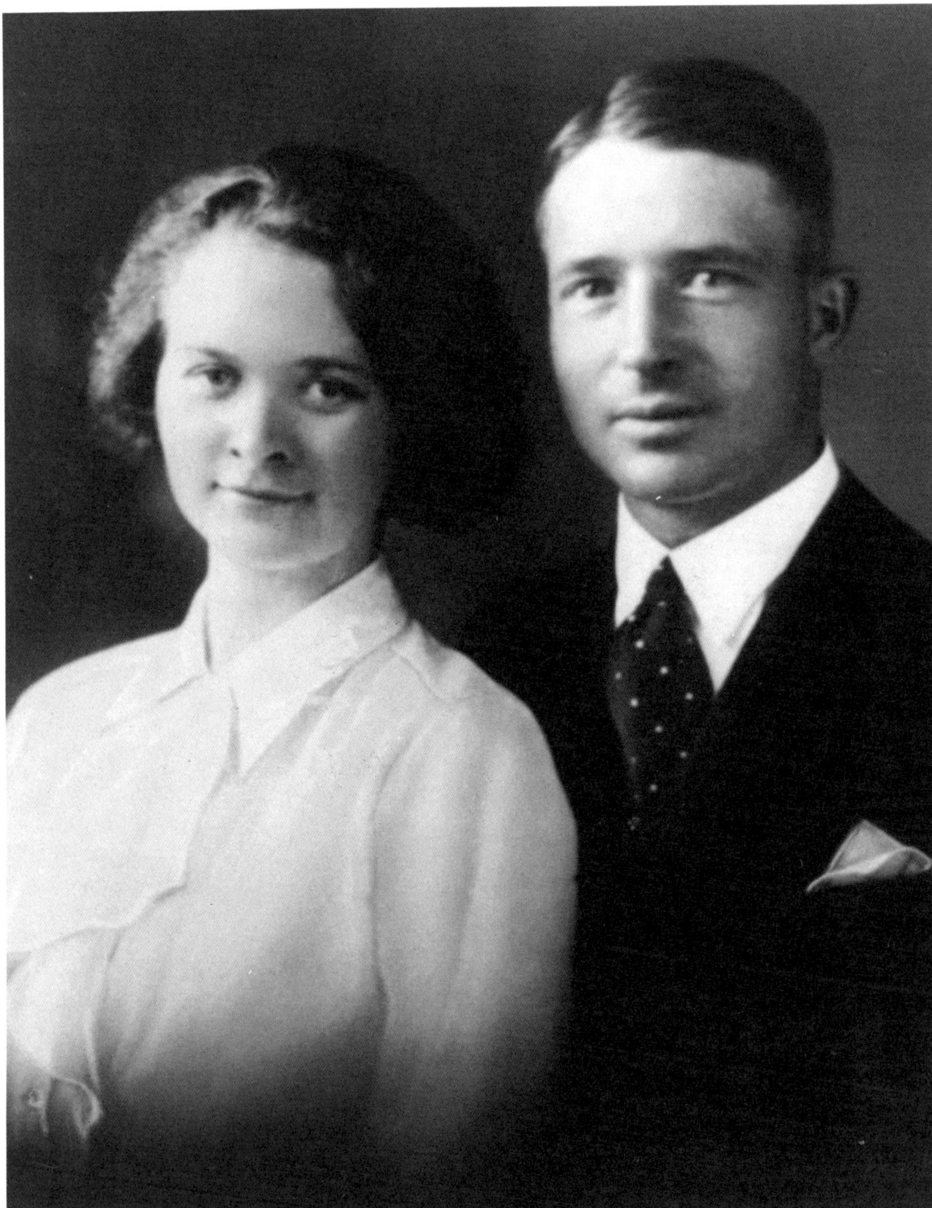

Wedding portrait of Theodore and Anna Hermesmeyer, my Mama and Papa.

I would like to take a moment to thank Mama and Papa for the unbelievable sacrifices they made trying to survive World War II with four children. As children we see things so differently—we are in our fantasy world. However, grownups do not have this luxury. Yes, the war was terrible for us children, but I now know that it was much worse for Mama and Papa. It is hard for me to even imagine my children having little clothing, going hungry or having their safety endangered. Yet, for my parents, this was a daily reality. They had to endure not only their own pain, but also that of their children.

Papa worked from four in the morning until ten in the evening almost every day to ensure that we would have something to wear and eat. Mama was ill much of the time, and the war took its toll on my parents' relationship. I wish to let my Mama and Papa know how much I appreciate everything they did for us.

I feel that Beyond The Dark Cloud *would not be complete without thanking my dear parents.*

I know that they are both in Heaven.

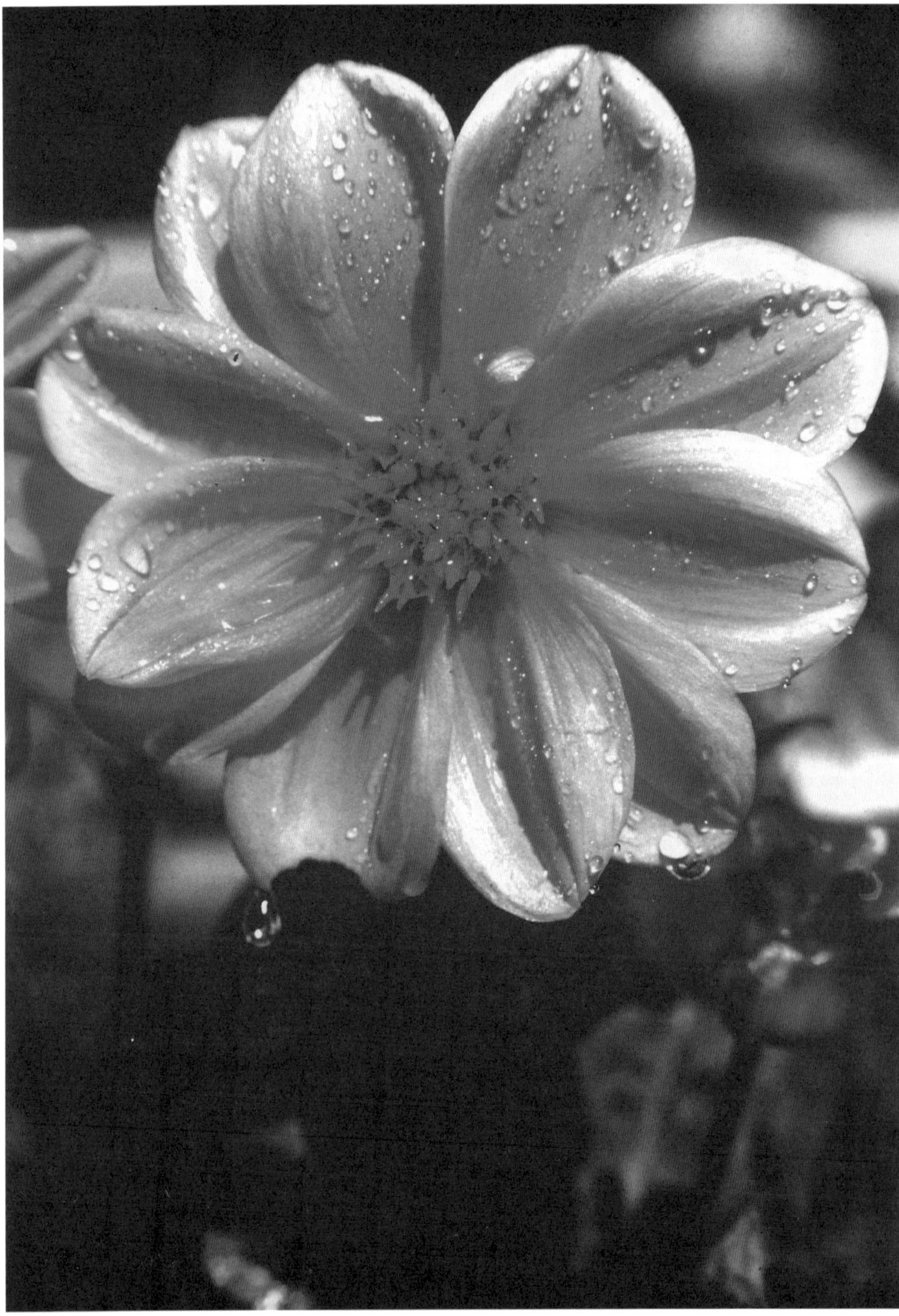

Photo by Thea.

My most sincere thank you and deepest appreciation to Eva Alvarez who typed Beyond The Dark Cloud. *Eva is an Environmental Law student at the University of California in Santa Barbara. I know that without Eva's dedication, this book would not be finished today.*

Eva, my friend,
I would like to dedicate this flower on the opposite page to you. You did such a beautiful job, thank you so much. You helped my dream become reality.

God Bless You, Eva

Thea

Table of Contents

Foreword

By Jay A Goldstein, M.D.

In this book, my patient Thea Schlosser describes her personal experiences with a frustrating illness that baffles physicians and the lay public alike. Like many afflicted individuals, Ms. Schlosser has endured financial and interpersonal deprivations from the ravages of her disorder, Chronic Fatigue and Immune Dysfunction.

She has tried to leave no stone unturned in her quest for understanding and treating her disabling symptoms, and shares her insights with the reader. Although her life has been almost ruined by her disease, she nevertheless retains an optimism and spirituality that are so important when dealing with chronic impairment. Her tribulations are variations on the consistent pattern of being labeled "lazy and crazy" that I have encountered in the thousands of patients I have treated. By describing these travails for the reader, the feeling of isolation that so many patients have could be ameliorated, and significant others in a patient's life may not be so prone to stigmatize an individual who had previously been healthy and vibrant.

Ms. Schlosser's therapeutic trials have been quite eclectic, and the results of her interactions with health care professionals are mixed with her personal views about the value of various remedies. She presents a cornucopia of treatment options, which are purely anecdotal, but may be of interest to like-minded individuals.

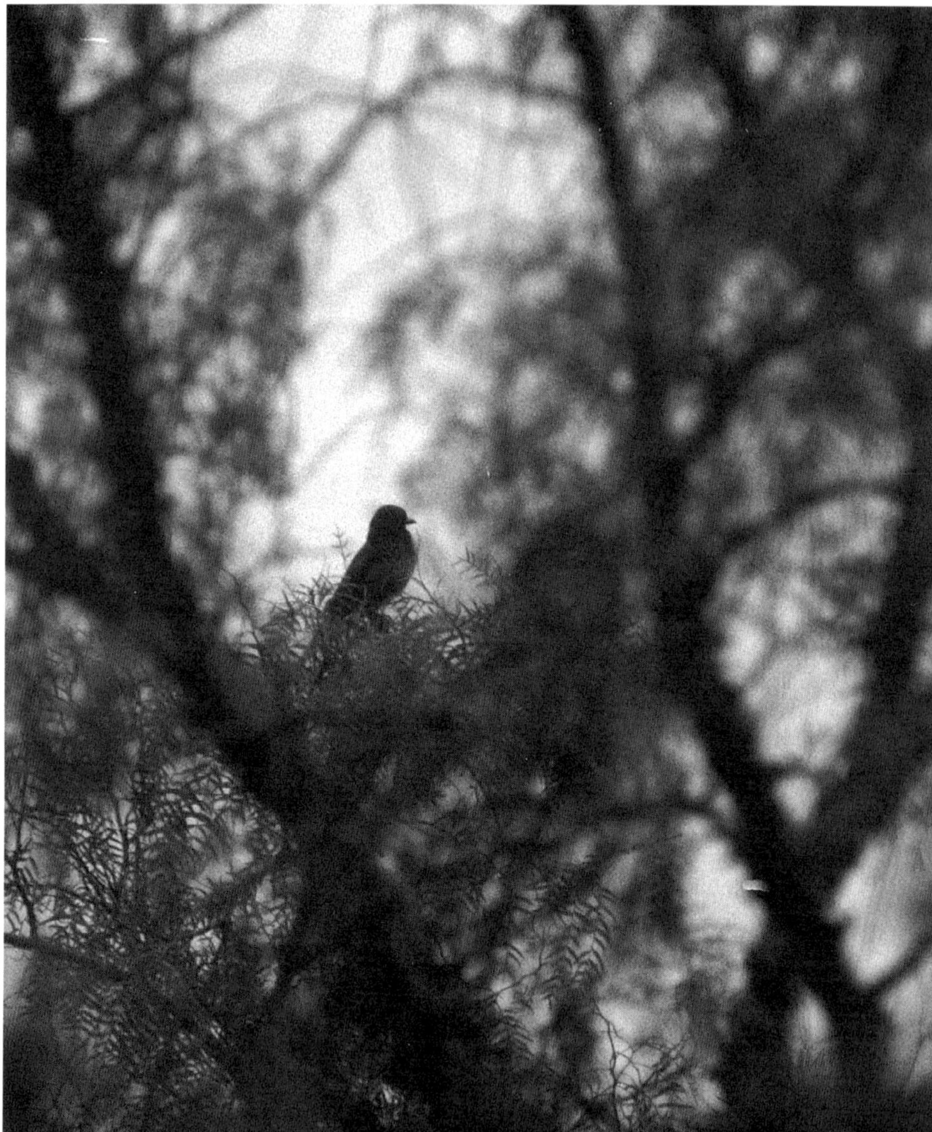

Photo by Thea.

Preface

By Lona Peoples

When I first met Thea, we spoke with each other about our lives, as new friends will do. We both sought to be heard and understood, and were thoughtful regarding each other's feelings.

She was recovering from a serious bout of encephalitis and Chronic Fatigue and, I, too, had for many years experienced a lot of the same symptoms, and had also remained a puzzlement to the medical establishment. I had finally, just that week, been diagnosed as a universal reactor with an immune system dysfunction. It was a short while later that the words chronic fatigue were added.

So I could relate very closely to many of her feelings of helplessness and frustrations at a modern medical model that had no place to put us and the fast-growing numbers of others like us.

Because of this common thread between us, we were mutually supportive, an important element in any friendship.

As she spoke of her life, her love for her daughters, her gratitude to them and to Karl for their love and support for her, I heard the caring in her voice. I also heard the grief of her losses, her deep and reverent belief in, faith in, and love for God, as well as her commitment to her healing and her life.

She talked of her desire to use her life and what she had learned through the years about her illness to help others find the pathway to healing as she was doing.

Showing so vividly through all her pain were memories of a childhood of fear and insecurity in war-torn Germany. Of bombs and fires. Of horror on the faces of her parents and other adults as they sought safety for themselves and their children where there was none to be found. Of hunger, thirst, darkness, cold, defeat, and despair of those around her. Of death and birth amidst rubble and ruin. Impossible situations where the will to survive was a constant and all-consuming struggle and, yet, a deep innate desire in all of them.

Finally came the end of the war, and a new kind of struggle began. One where life was restored to some kind of order and balance and young Thea grew older with the passing of time.

Through the years that we have been friends, Thea has spoken to me of a different era in her life and the creeping through her of this unknown illness, stalking her body. A phantom that no one could see, pulling her away from activity and from her very existence. The years of no diagnosis, of misdiagnosis, and of no or wrong medical and psychological evaluations and treatment, as she pled to be heard, to find help.

With each new physician was the added hope that maybe this one would hear her, would know what to do to help end the extreme fatigue, increasing muscle pain and weakness, debilitating headaches, inability to perform neither the simple nor the complex tasks of homemaking and managing her photography business or to attend functions. She had done all these things and more so effortlessly before.

I have learned more about her life and her losses, which have continued to occur because of this illness. Through it all, an image began to take form in my mind, and I knew that **her story must be told, must be written, and that it must become alive with motion through the media of film,** so that others like her may **recognize themselves** and **understand that there is a way to heal.**

For Thea has indeed emerged from behind a dark cloud, from many dark clouds. She has come forth with a message **of renewed hope** and courage and the promise to others that the same thing can happen to them. Because she has been there and returned, she offers to show them the way.

Thea is a heroine in an era where there are few of them. She is a woman who can be an example for others who are ill and lonely with rejection and abandonment and struggle to survive.

It is my plea to all those who have misunderstood her symptoms and ours: Please, please, for the sake of all humanity in this age, listen to those who seek your help. Hear us all, and never, never, never say, "It's all in your head."

Thank you, Thea, for being a voice for all of us. Perhaps because of your willingness to share your story so openly and with such honesty and courage, more medical, professional, clergy, and family members and others will hear our cry. For it is, after all, their cry, too. As it was Dante's cry, echoing down eternity's chasms, beseeching, "Do not forsake me, do not leave me. Stand by me now in heart's plight. Do not leave me to suffer in this underworld alone."

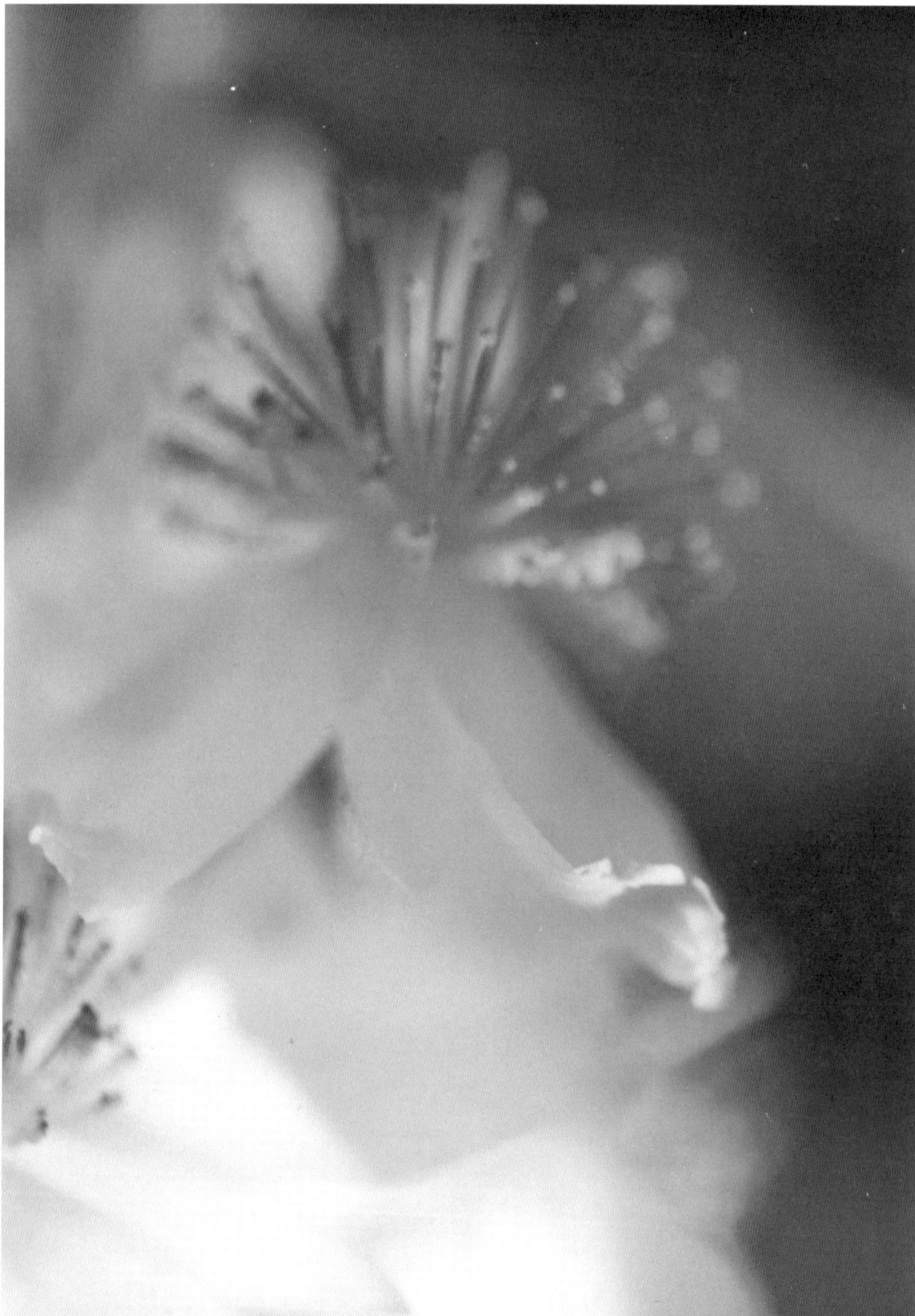

Photo by Thea.

Introduction

BY PROFESSOR WOLFRAM KÜHNAU, M.D.

The special value of this moving book lies in the fact that it is utterly devoid of the slightest indication of artificiality, sensation mongering, or personal vanity. The author's narrative is genuine, clear, and taken from pure experience, which makes the book all the more valuable and believable. From a literary point of view, this is a particularly happy circumstance! The reader senses from the very first few lines how much anguish and humiliation the author had to go through while never losing faith in finally triumphing over her illness. This book is also irreplaceable as a form of documentation. The portrayal of symptoms and the discouraging remarks by physicians, that nothing much could possibly be done in any case, make it plausible that a person would ultimately have to give up in utter despair and consider suicide as the only solution. The book demonstrates beautifully that it should never come to that, and therein lies its great value. The gloomy background to it is constituted by the incredible arrogance and superciliousness of a dehumanized "orthodox" practice of medicine that sees its highest goal in the cataloguing of illnesses while totally ignoring human dignity. This disregard for human needs leads to an utter disavowal of the Hippocratic Oath.

The physician is the "apparatchnick," as the Russians express it appropriately: a ruthless, computer-like way of thinking. This leads to an indiscriminate esteem in which laboratory medicine scoffs at medical experience that has been gathered through the millennia. All of this makes up the bitter background of this excellent book, which fearlessly uncovers such faulty thinking.

I am thinking in this context of my neighbor who felt that he could afford early retirement and planned to tend his garden. While still in his early sixties, he suddenly displayed the classic symptoms of angina pectoris and rushed himself to the closest American University Clinic. A fully computerized exam declared him to be in perfect health and saw no reason for concern. He died the next day upon his return home. A classic death caused by heart disease! It turns out that the most important part of the exam had been omitted because it was deemed "old-fashioned." This is the exam by auscultation and percussion: the simple listening to the heart and tapping of the chest! Christian Morgenstern formulated this very appropriately. He concluded crystal clear that, "nothing will exist that is not allowed to exist."

Just because I do not have the proper instruments to diagnose an illness at my disposal does not mean that the illness simply does not exist! This is the point that the book brings home. In 1983 there was a Chronic Fatigue epidemic in Lake Tahoe. Suddenly there *was* an illness after all, and *now* the finer instruments were going to be applied. Instead of a case of "pater peccavi" as in traditional medicine, the race was now on for the presumable virus that eludes us to this day. And now one begins to realize at long last that the origins of all evil lay in a malfunction of the body, that is, of the immune system.

We should let the author speak in her own words, of course. I think, though, that the reader will learn rather quickly that here is a document which can only be compared to "Simplicius Simplicissimus" by Gimmelshausen, who portrayed in an innocent, childlike manner all of the untold and unimaginable sufferings of the Thirty Years War. This book has a similar kind of immediacy that ought to put all those learned physicians to shame. If it could convince our arrogant physicians that it is finally time for self-reflection, then, apart from all that is so utterly humane in it, this book will become an everlasting milestone in the history of medicine.

Prologue

When I made my decision to write this book in 1990, I knew it would be a challenge. But life is filled with challenges. I have started to write this book many times during the past six years, but as many of you know all too well, CFIDS is so unpredictable, one must wait for the moment when you feel better and have a vision of what you want to do. One has to wait for that time when the brain feels less painful and foggy and when the pain coursing through the body is less intense, as it is never completely gone. It truly feels like an impossible dream to realize that I have finally completed this book. As a survivor of CFIDS, I know all too well that simple tasks like going to the supermarket or taking a shower, or even brushing your teeth, can be major undertakings.

When I first started this book, I thought that just sharing my uphill battle with CFIDS would be enough. But then I realized that I wanted to help those who are struggling with CFIDS as I am, from a nutritional, physical, emotional, and spiritual point of view. In order to do this, I have included a section describing some of the most common symptoms of CFIDS, as well as sections with possible ways to cope with this disease and inspiring poems. There are also sections outlining some of the treatments and supplements available to those suffering from CFIDS. The last section includes a variety of articles on CFIDS-related topics written by experts in this area.

I tried my best to put a book together that would share my life with you. None of us who endure CFIDS must ever give up hope or think less about ourselves. Although we have an illness that virtually owns our entire bodies and our entire lives, there is always light at the end of the tunnel. I wish to share with you how I survived a nightmare almost beyond my ability to comprehend. It is a story of a desperate struggle to have this disease properly diagnosed and taken care of. It is a story of grief, pain, medical misdiagnosis, and recovery. My journey through the nightmare of CFIDS sent me from having a loving family and being a successful and well-respected businesswoman, enjoying complete financial security, all the way down to the bottom. I lost the most important thing of all: my ability to be a functioning, loving, caring mother and wife. All of these things were torn away from me because of my catastrophic breakdown.

Chapter One

A Brief Account of My Life and Personal Battle with CFIDS

Childhood: WW II and Molestation

I was raised in Germany during World War II. Prior to the war, my family was financially secure, and we enjoyed a fine standard of living. I grew up with one brother, Hugo, and two sisters, Maria and Anneliese. My childhood during the war years was dramatic. I had known deprivation, hardship, psychological abuse, molestation, and fear.

I vividly remember working in a coal mine during the war at the age of eight. I washed floors and ran errands to help my family to try to survive. We combed our hair with a fork for a long time, because we had no comb or brush, and we could not afford to buy one. Sometimes, we had no shoes to wear. For years, our food consisted of bean soup. The war was a traumatic experience. Menaced continuously by military attacks, we never knew if and when the next bomb would hit us or tear our family apart. Living for years in terror cannot be described in words. Fear and hunger became a way of life. Then one day the fighting stopped, and we realized that somehow, by a miracle, we had survived.

One of my saddest memories from childhood is molestation. I was so afraid to tell anyone and ashamed. It happened with a neighbor. He touched and fondled me. Once you are molested, your self-worth is almost non-existent, leaving the door open for this terrible crime to be repeated. I wanted to tell my Mama what had happened to me. One day I finally got enough courage to approach her as she was

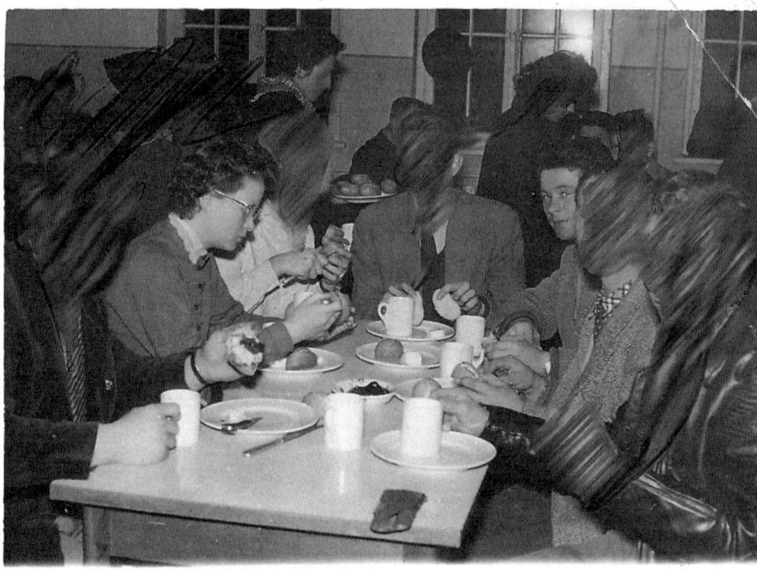

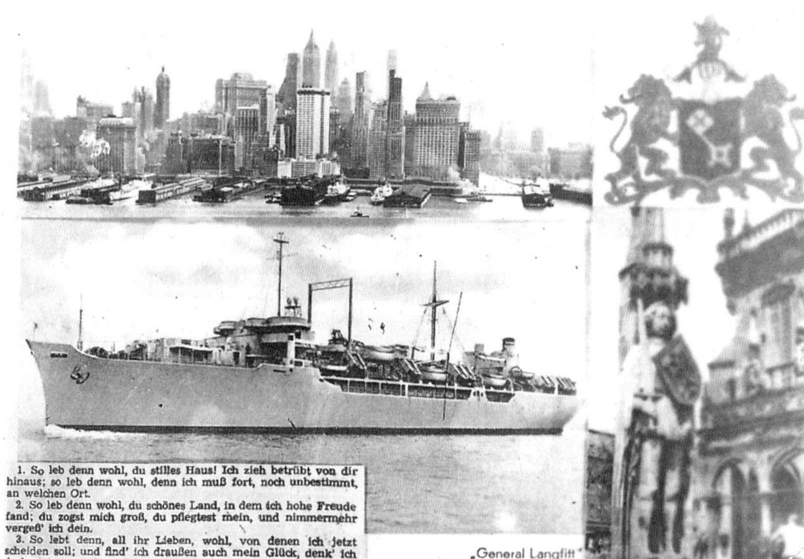
1. So leb denn wohl, du stilles Haus! Ich zieh betrübt von dir hinaus; so leb denn wohl, denn ich muß fort, noch unbestimmt, an welchen Ort.
2. So leb denn wohl, du schönes Land, in dem ich hohe Freude fand; du zogst mich groß, du pflegtest mein, und nimmermehr vergeß' ich dein.
3. So lebt denn, all ihr Lieben, wohl, von denen ich jetzt scheiden soll; und find' ich draußen auch mein Glück, denk' ich doch stets an euch zurück.
„General Langfitt"

Karl and I arrived in New York in 1956 on this boat. My eyes opened with joy as I saw the majestic Statue of Liberty.

talking to my sister Maria. As I got closer, she began screaming that she was going to go to the police. This scared me. Maria was telling Mama that the neighbor who had molested me had tried unsuccessfully to molest her. I was sure that if I told my mother about this that she would inform the police and that I would go to prison. Needless to say, a child is never at **fault!**

I had to learn to love, care, and respect myself again. This took a lot of time. We all have a child inside of us. Every once in a while, I embrace "Little Thea" and give her comfort, love, compassion, and, most of all, a safe place. I know this sounds a little corny, but it works. Unless we heal the wounded child in us, we cannot heal our bodies and minds. It is impossible to forget such a dramatic experience, but we need to forgive, and this can be accomplished with time.

Despite my difficult childhood, I became the national freestyle swimming champion of Austria in 1950. I also managed to become a ping pong champion and an accomplished skier. At the same time, I developed my passion for writing and art.

Immigrating from Austria to Beautiful America

At the age of eighteen, I married my former childhood friend, Karl Schlosser. Shortly after that, in 1956, we emigrated to America. We traveled on a military ship. I will never forget what it meant to us to see the Statue of Liberty; what a sense of freedom. We found a new beginning, with new possibilities, that no other country could offer us at that point.

As we moved on to Los Angeles, it seemed like we were living in a fairy tale. We could hardly believe the unexpected comfort that existed at that time in the United States. What a joy to wash ourselves with hot and cold water coming directly from the tap. No more going to the water well two or three times a day just to fetch water, no matter what the weather was. Shopping in a supermarket and discovering the rich variety of food was just unbelievable for me. I was very impressed with how helpful the American people were to us. I was so touched by the comfort and love offered to us that I wanted to have all of my family with me, to share my experience, especially my mother.

Our beginning in the United States was a tremendous challenge.

We did not speak the English language, we had no money, and I was pregnant. During our first years here, Karl worked very hard for the family, putting in many hours of overtime. In order to survive, we had to work various jobs.

Karl had begun drinking in Austria. Although he did not drink often, when he did drink, he drank to the point of "blacking out." Now, in the United States, his "blackouts" were becoming more frequent as his ambitions to reach his highest goals for the family drove him to drinking more often.

In 1957, our beautiful daughter Ingrid was born. What a bundle of joy! Sadly, five months later, I received a letter that my mother had died. Mama had been very sick in Austria for years. She suffered from seriously ulcerated legs and from a severe form of hypothyroid disease for which there was no treatment available at the time. Hypothyroidism has many symptoms, one of which is severe depression. Mama committed suicide at the age of 46. This was a tremendous loss. I felt as if my whole world had collapsed.

When I received the news of my mother's death, Ingrid was only five months old. Adding to all of this the fact that I was living in a foreign country, not knowing the language, brought to me, all of a sudden, the shadow side of our fairy tale.

Intellectually, my mother was about 20 years ahead of her time, and because of this, there were many people who did not understand her. Early in my life, noticed a gift Mama possessed. She had the ability to ease other people's pain and to love unconditionally. This made my mother an incredible person. I had always been very close to her. I miss her very much.

At the same time that I received the bad news about my mother, I found that I was pregnant with our second daughter Evelyn, whom we call Elly. Although I had lost my mother, God blessed us with another precious child.

We did everything we could to provide a beautiful childhood for our children. They received piano lessons and accordion lessons. They went to a German and Catholic school and belonged to a German band. We tried to raise our children with a lot of love and understanding. We tried to treat them as people, without much judgment, encouraging their sense of self, helping to develop their self-confidence, a sense of faith, trust in themselves and in others, a sense of honesty, responsibility, and self-respect. The children learned to appreciate what they had, rather than regret what they did not have. There was mutual trust and consideration. I am quite certain that we made plenty of mistakes raising our little angels, but we gave it our best shot.

First Sign of CFIDS

Everything seemed to be perfect. A good future seemed to appear on the horizon for the children and ourselves. Then, in 1970, I had this overwhelming feeling of exhaustion starting all of a sudden. Like during the war, a bomb had hit, but this time it was a different bomb, and a **new battle began.** It began with **mononucleosis,** which was exhausting. As I became more and more ill, our children no longer enjoyed a normal, carefree childhood. I needed help with the household, driving became difficult, and cooking less frequent. Reading a story to Ingrid and Elly or doing homework with them became nearly impossible. I kept thinking, "What is wrong with me?"

While battling mononucleosis, I received the horrible news that Papa had been diagnosed with lung cancer. He, too, committed suicide. Now I had to face the fact that both of my parents were no longer with me. I felt horribly guilty over their deaths. I often asked myself if I could have saved them by not leaving Austria. Did I desert them? It took me a long time to get over my feelings of guilt, but I now know that their deaths were not my fault.

I never fully regained my strength after my bout with mononucleosis. I never felt the "same" again. Regardless of how much rest or sleep I got, I felt sick. It was a terrible, frightening experience to first realize that my mind was not working the same way as it used to.

I realized that I could not always control my moods. I felt confused, anxious, and depressed. I had no energy at all. I began to have night sweats, headaches, general body pain, and one infection after another. The doctors tried antibiotics. I had bouts of sinusitis that ultimately resulted in nine surgeries. I had tonsillitis so many times that the infections actually destroyed all of my tonsil tissue!

By early 1971, I had become so ill that my regular doctor was unable to help me. Unable to discover any serious physical problem, he felt that I had to be sent to a psychiatrist to be treated for depression. The psychiatrist suggested hospitalization. I was so despaired about the thought of my children being without me that I decided there was absolutely no way that I would enter the psychiatric hospital. However, my illness soon got to the point where I felt totally helpless. Finally I had no choice, I had to go, no matter how terrible I felt about it.

I still remember one of the first patients I met. She had virtually the same symptoms as I had. She had also lost her business, a beauty salon. She had been hospitalized for months, and yet she acted so "normal" in comparison to the other patients. Neither of us could figure out why we were so exhausted all of the time, so tired, so sick. Neither could the medical professionals.

Electric Shock Treatments

It was finally suggested that we receive electric shock treatments. As scared as I was, I wanted to get better again and hoped that the treatment would be beneficial. Both of us were given the "full course." Electric shock treatments then were much different than they are now.

I clearly remember waiting in a room with about 12 patients for our shock treatments. Not only did we have to wait until our turn, but we had to endure the anxiety and fear of seeing the patients who went in for treatment ahead of us being brought back out again. Keep in mind that this was 1971. These poor souls would come staggering out, dazed and confused, looking like they had been hit over the head with a mallet. It was a horrible, frightening sight, made incalculably worse by the fact that my turn was coming quite soon.

After being in the hospital for one month, and having received five or six electric shock treatments, I had lost 28 pounds. My memory and all of my pre-existing symptoms got worse. Reality almost began to dissolve, and I did not know anymore what was really happening. I no longer felt human. I felt scared and dazed.

These "treatments" actually seemed to help a small number of the patients receiving them: those truly suffering from some neurological or psychological disorder that apparently was treatable with this "medical technique." Sadly, each treatment made my condition worse. By 1973, I had received 19 electric shock treatments for an undiagnosed disease. At this point, my husband refused to allow the doctors to continue treatment. I was in and out of the hospital regularly, and still no one could find out what was wrong with me. **NO ONE.** I was finally released in 1973, but not for long.

I quickly found myself back in the mental ward of the hospital being attended by a new psychiatrist. Realizing that I really did have a sinus infection, she sent me to an ear, nose, and throat specialist who confirmed my condition and put me on MORE antibiotics. I spent the next nine months in the mental ward, taking antibiotics. My eyes were continually bloodshot, and I had massive sinus headaches. Through all of this, I was essentially bedridden. I worried about my precious children and about my husband Karl all the time. My family came to see me often.

My sister Anneliese would come to see me often and turned me over, because I had developed severe bed sores. She convinced me to see a different ear, nose, and throat specialist, who told us that I needed an immediate sinus operation. My infection was out of control by this time, and my life was in danger. This difficult procedure was performed in a regular hospital. The amount of congealed and hardened green puss in my frontal sinuses alone equaled two golf balls in size, and they had to be scraped from the bones of my skull. Tonsil tools, not sinus tools, had to be employed because the infection was so far out of control. The doctor said after the surgery, "Thea, you were as close to death as anyone can get. You do not belong in a mental ward." He was surprised that I could have possibly gone through all these days, weeks, and months with such a massive infection.

I spent five days in a regular hospital after the surgery and then four days in the mental ward. I was then discharged. My sinuses were continually drained and treated both in the hospital and in the doctor's office. The sinus surgery relieved some of the pain, but it was not the answer to all of my symptoms.

My ear, nose, and throat specialist advised me to see an endocrinologist. He discovered a cyst on my thyroid, which had to be removed. Hypothyroidism runs in our family. My mother suffered from it in an extreme case, and my sister Anneliese, as well as my daughter Ingrid, are also affected by it. I knew I was quite ill, but I could not quite put my finger on the possible cause; neither could the medical profession.

November 6, 1974

Re: Dorothea B. Schlosser

It is my understanding that the insurance file for Mrs. Dorothea B. Schlosser is presently under your supervision.

Mrs. Schlosser was a patient at Compton Foundation Hospital from October 22, 1973 to December 3, 1973. She has been a patient at this hospital from March 29, 1974 to and including the present time. The diagnosis of this patient's illness has consistently been as follows: (1) Anxiety neurosis, (2) Hypoglycemia, (3) Chronic sinusitis.

The diagnosis of anxiety neurosis was given first because this is essentially a psychiatric hospital. However, there seems no question from the standpoint of the clinical history of this patient that the anxiety which she subsequently suffered was triggered by a very severe attack of hypoglycemia undiagnosed at the time, later coming into considerable investigative consideration of organic brain pathology.

During this patient's hospital stay as part of the routine diagnostic procedures, she was given a 5-hour glucose tolerance test. The results of this test were confirmatory and most specifically of the hypoglycemic diagnosis. Since the symptoms of the hypoglycemic state itself are often confused with those of depressive and anxiety neuroses, being very similar both objectively and subjectively, it is understandable why, after the likelihood of organic brain pathology was ruled out, this patient came under primary psychiatric consideration. The long period of doubt as to the proper diagnosis, the unsuccessful psychiatric approach, each in itself would tend to create anxiety in the average individual.

It is the opinion of the writer, from the vantage point of laboratory findings and long clinical observation, that undoubtedly the patient's primary problem was a physical problem and that hypoglycemia suggested by the chronic sinusitis resulted in anxiety both as part of the hypoglycemic reactions and consequent to them.

It is your client's understanding that insurance benefits for physically-based illness are more flexible and of more lengthy duration than those based primarily on psychiatric illnesses. If this is true, it would be a logical assumption that Mrs. Schlosser's case justifies review from the standpoint of insurance benefits.

Should this letter be addressed to persons other than yourself, perhaps you would be kind enough to arrange for its proper destination. Thank you for whatever you are able to do to assist Mrs. Schlosser in regard to her insurance difficulties.

Very truly yours,
Assistant Medical Director

Letter to insurance company.

At one point, I was given a hypoglycemia test. The results of the hourly readings were 48 (before the glucose) and 105, 150, 33, 195, and 65 after the glucose. The massive drop between the third and fourth hour was simply more than my body could handle, and I went into a seizure.

Exhaustion and Pain

My fatigue or, more correctly, my exhaustion went on uninterrupted. My frustration grew daily as I visited medical doctor after doctor and chiropractor after chiropractor. I attended health forums, read volumes of articles and books, and spent countless hours talking to people on the phone, hoping somehow to find a clue as to what was happening to my life energy. As early as 1974, I began taking massive vitamin and nutritional therapy. I was "eating right" and trying to "think positively," but nothing could reverse the overwhelming, never-ending exhaustion. I even went to health spas on occasion and tried to go to bed early each night, hoping that I would have a little more energy during the next day. Nothing worked. I have always been an achiever, but this disease took all of my life energy away. For a period of six years, electric shock treatments, tranquilizers, antidepressants, and painkillers made my health condition worse. I was so tired that I could not even watch TV.

I was also subject to unexplainable headaches, which would strike at any moment. Some were so severe that I wanted to scream. I would sometimes get just enough energy to go out briefly and drive somewhere; unfortunately, I felt "lost," disoriented, and unable to make sense of the traffic lights. Most of the time, the kids would head off to school, and I would just go back to bed and collapse.

In 1974, we moved from Los Angeles to Santa Barbara, a distance of about 100 miles. The move was very rough on all of us. Karl and I started a metal fabrication business. At first it was a challenge, but I had all the faith in the world in Karl. I underwent dramatic weight loss and endured another sinus surgery, not nearly as bad as the first procedure, but very difficult nevertheless.

I began to notice that my mystery disease started to take on new characteristics. Now I had virtually no tolerance for noise. Household noises were the most common source of discomfort. Sometimes

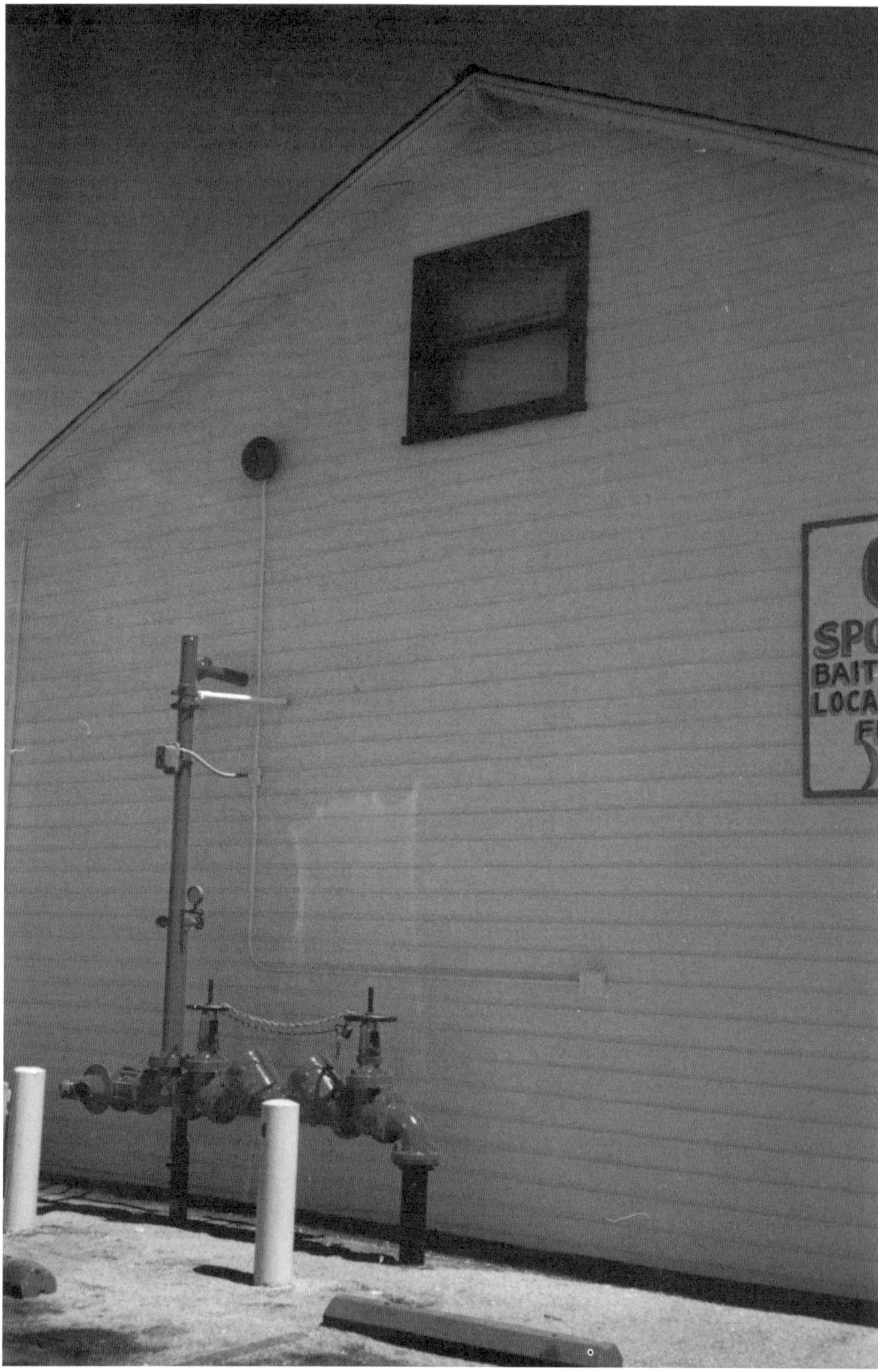

Photo by Thea.

I often rested in one of our closets just to reduce the noise level. I even wore noise reducers, similar to those worn by construction workers. They hurt my head, but it was better than having to listen to the television or to the phone ringing.

According to the doctors, my physical exhaustion and emotional confusion were "in my head." I continuously asked myself: Why am I sick all the time? Why all this emotional and physical exhaustion? Why all the infections?

Since I could not go out much most of the time, photography became a favorite hobby. I began to take pictures around the house and sometimes out the windows. I never was a painter or musician, but I had always been touched and inspired by beauty and art. It has always been a wonderful experience for me to capture beauty by making photographs. I could still see life's beauty all around me through my camera lens. Capturing a flower's beauty re-awakened me to life and filled my heart and soul with joy. Creating was a challenge, but also a great satisfaction. The excitement of discovering great results increased my sense of self-worth. Soon, I was actually able to sell some of my photographs.

Isn't it magical to be able to discover the sometimes hidden beauty of the universe, of our environment, or of a situation? Energy low, body pain, swollen glands, nightsweats, headache and so on—I was desperate—desperate to do something.

1977: My Own Camera Store

Somehow in 1977, and only God knows how, I came up with the idea that I should open a camera business. I felt capable of running a small business in photography and camera sales, if I could plan everything in detail and take care of my energy and household. So, with only my own camera and lens, and a burning desire, I started my own used camera and mail order business.

Frankly, one of the *prime motivations* behind my business venture was to somehow earn some **respect** from the medical profession, which had, for years, been suggesting that my illness was **"all in my head."** I sadly found out that once you are diagnosed as emotionally ill, the doctors will *always* treat you differently. Worse yet, they typecast you, labeling you as "emotionally ill" forever, whether you're really ill or not.

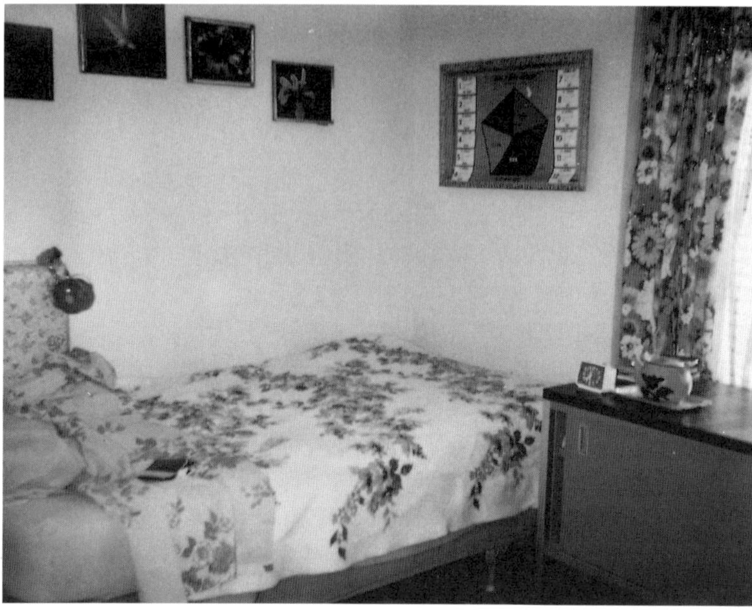

I started my mail order camera business from my home so that I could rest whenever I needed to.

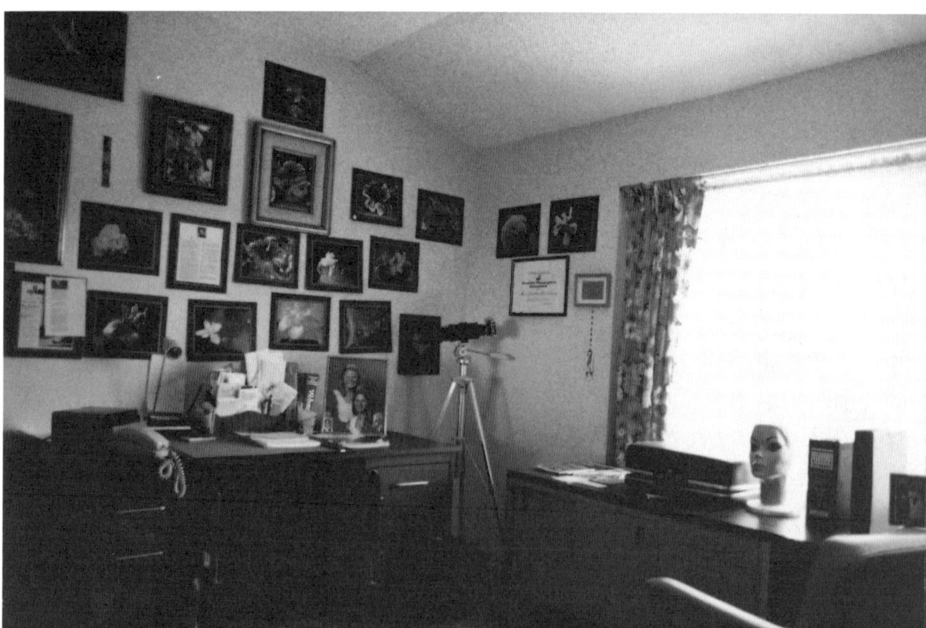

As my business grew, all I had was my camera, some photographs, an answering machine, will power, and a lot of patience.

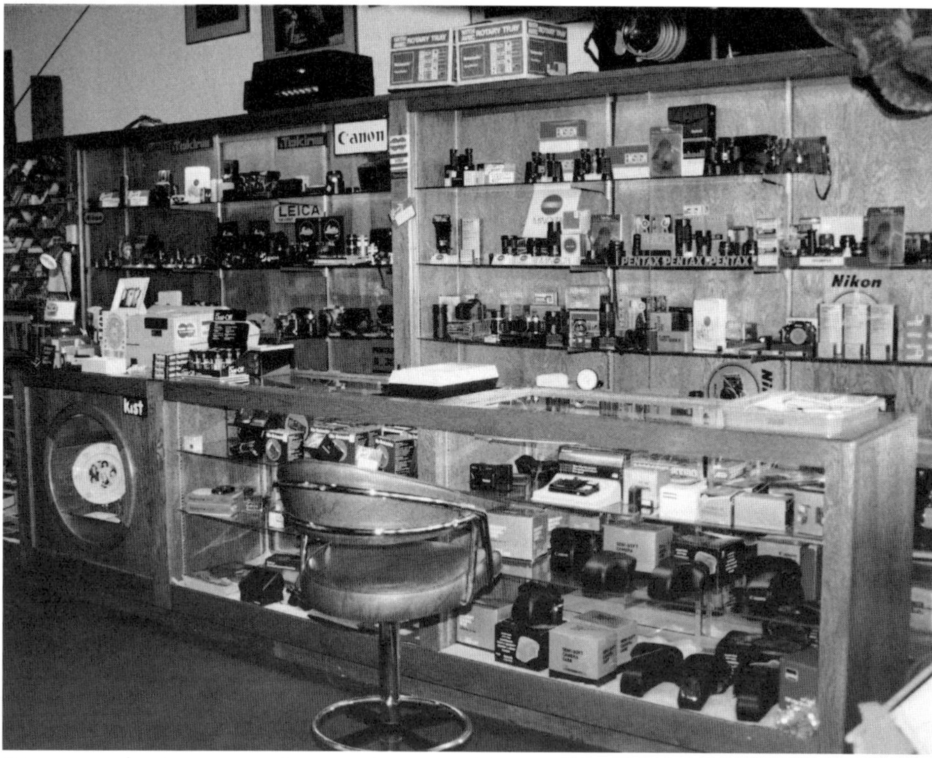

My camera business grew from my home to this store located in a shopping mall in Santa Barbara. I had the joy and pleasure of designing the display shelves shown above. They were custom-made.

New doctors would take the advice of previous doctors, and I found myself on a merry-go-round, almost in the way a criminal is always labeled as a criminal. This is wrong. **VERY WRONG!**

I realized that the success or failure of my business would ultimately measure my success as a human being. I find this both **unfair** and **sad,** but it is the **reality.**

I had only two hundred and fifty dollars that was left of my inheritance from my parents' estate as startup money. I had no camera retail experience. I was even too tired to drive myself to the State Board of Equalization Office to apply for my retail business license and had to ask a friend to drive me there. Still, I wanted to start my own business. I took things one step at a time. Baby steps.

I began by working out of my home. Because I did not always have the energy to talk, the first thing I did was to get an answering machine. This way, I could return calls when I was able to. For the first seven months, my only partner was my answering machine. I soon hired my daughter Elly and made her a 50% partner. Elly learned this difficult business quickly, and my customers really liked her. To this day, I so much appreciate her efforts. Elly began to take care of the customers' calls from nine to five, six days a week.

I had to make the money last, so advertising was very important. I started with some small ads in the internationally circulated "Shutterbug," a magazine for those interested in purchasing and selling photographic equipment. I took cameras and equipment on consignment and tried to sell them. I charged only 10% as a consignment fee and worked myself, painfully and slowly, to the position of a respected businesswoman with an ever-growing love for photography and people. I learned an incredible amount, both about people and about the retail business.

That first year, although I continued to fight my unknown illness, I sold about $7,000 worth of used cameras. I was ecstatic. I was then able to rent a small retail store front and go "legitimate." My second year, sales soared to more than $64,000, the third year to $130,000, and the fourth up to an incredible $300,000! I was fortunate to receive two nationwide write-ups regarding my accomplishments, which gave me a great sense of satisfaction. I was then given the great honor of being voted into the "Who's Who In American Business Women." Then, in 1984, I was nominated and inducted into the prestigious "Foremost Women of the Twentieth Century." I felt extremely honored and happy.

It seemed that, as my business success grew, so did the power of my unknown illness. However, my desire to make my business a success, along with the love and help of my daughter and loyal staff, enabled me to achieve what I did.

Unfortunately, my neck pain was increasing. There were many times when I could not go to work at all. The night sweats, headaches, and muscle pains were almost unbearable, but although I was drowning more into my disease, I persevered. Finally, I went to my current doctor and explained the story I had already told so many other doctors. Being a general practitioner and a psychiatrist, he treated me for depression and put me on antidepressants and tranquilizers. Nothing helped. As I reached the pinnacle of success as a businesswoman, my disease controlled me more powerfully than ever. By this time, I had found an excellent new location for my camera store and was able to buy my own photolab, thanks to my husband Karl.

In 1984, I was involved in a freak accident. While preparing for a garage sale, I opened a cabinet in my garage and a fifteen-pound steel transformer fell on the left side of my head. Even though I felt dizzy and nauseated, I did not seek immediate medical care, due to a previous commitment. Three days later, as the dizziness and discomfort continued to increase, I realized that I had to have medical attention and drove myself to the doctor's office. During my visit, I collapsed, and the physician's wife drove me to the hospital. I remained under treatment and observation for a severe concussion over the next two weeks.

That year saw me more at home than at work. My manager and daughter Elly would call for advice, which I would give over the telephone. I began to have trouble understanding how to run my own cash register; the numbers at times were just meaningless symbols. I couldn't even do credit card authorizations, because they were too confusing at times. I had my employees do them for me, although they did not know why. I was too embarrassed to explain that it was actually mentally painful and stressful. Putting numbers together made no sense, and that scared me. But still I kept smiling and talking and trying to carry on.

Doing my own TV and radio commercials was more and more difficult to do. My memory and my concentration got worse. I did not know how much longer I could put up a good front when, in reality, I felt as if I were dying. I had achieved so much, but now everything was beginning to crumble. Not being able to take care of my family was the most devastating for me.

My poor business. I had worked so hard to build it. "The castle that Thea built." I tried with all my heart to hold on to my store, but it was irrevocably slipping away.

My husband Karl had, during all this time, taken a very active role both in the household and at the store. At home he helped me cook, clean, do the laundry. and many other things to try to "keep the ship afloat." In the store, he also helped me greatly. Because my business grew so fast, it was very costly to keep a good stock of equipment. Karl helped me finance my store.

Because of Karl's long-time use of alcohol, we started family counseling. But Karl didn't feel it important enough to continue our sessions. The truth is, he did not want to stop drinking. According to the therapist, the best option for both of us was a divorce because, under these circumstances, our relationship would not improve and my health could only get worse. Karl was able to stop drinking for seven years, but in 1984 he had a business setback and started again.

My business, which had come to mean so much to me financially and symbolically, was now doomed. All the years of sweat and dedication were now disappearing before my eyes because of this horrible phantom illness. All the loving effort and support from Karl, our children, and my wonderful loyal customers could not stop my disease from invading me more and more.

I remember that particular day in 1984 as if it were yesterday. I walked into my store, called my loyal staff of six together, and told them that I was closing the business. Everybody was in shock. I felt as if someone had just cut off a part of my body. I walked out of the store, tears pouring down my face. I could not stop crying even while I was driving home. But I was thankful to God that I had the store as long as I did. I miss my store to this very day.

That was how it happened. And that was the end of practically everything. The unseen monster had consumed the last of my strength and energy.

Christmas 1985

By now, my divorce to Karl was almost final. My entire family, except me, went to Austria for Christmas. The symptoms then were so bad, and remained totally elusive to the medical community, that I actually began to believe that what they were telling me was true. I actually began to believe that my illness was a psychological disorder, nothing more, and that it was "all in my head."

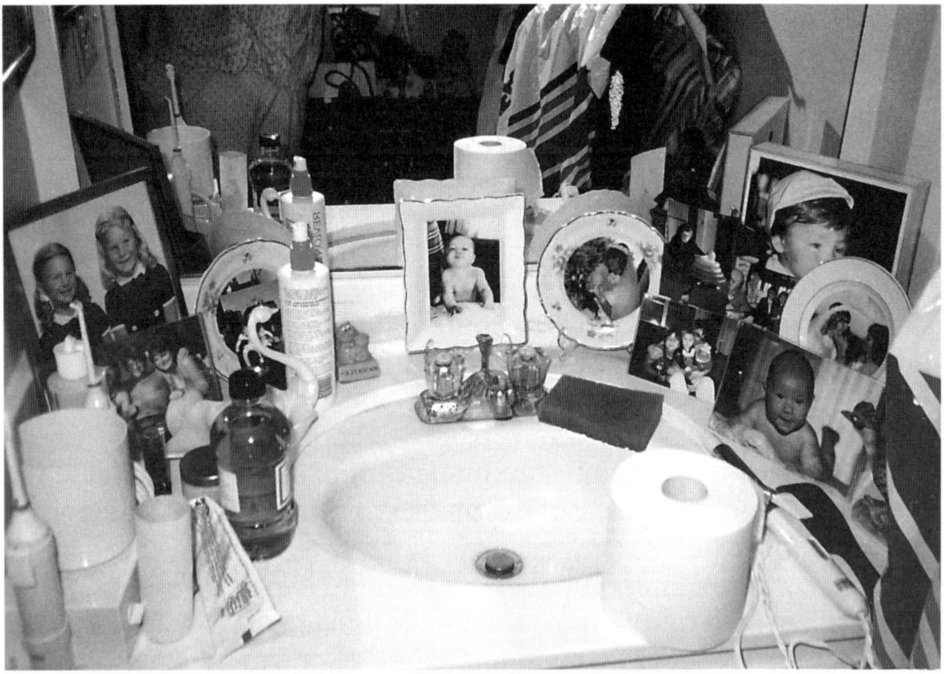

There was a time in 1985 when someone took me into her home. My space was very limited, so I used the sink counter to display photographs of my family.

During the entire year of 1985, I was in such mental and physical agony that I was given Ativan, a drug similar to Valium. As much as it helped numb my senses, it made me feel more like a zombie, and I quickly became addicted to it. This was completely unacceptable to me. I decided to get off the drug at once, and this was, of course, a big mistake. It is a must to withdraw from a drug dependency slowly. I became so sick just before Christmas that my neighbor had to drive me to the hospital. I was barely admitted when I began to have major seizures. The next day, I was told that I would have to pay five hundred dollars per day. Regardless of the seizures, I decided to take the risk and walk home since my home was very close to the hospital. I knew my insurance would not pay, and I could not afford to pay the five hundred dollars a day. I still remember walking in this horrible state of isolation.

I was only home a few minutes before the hospital staff, worried about my condition, sent an ambulance to my house and picked me up! They felt that further treatment was necessary. My withdrawal from Ativan created new symptoms and more pain. The hospital staff decided that it was not in my best interest to be alone at home, and they were right. They transferred me to the mental ward. Having been out of mental wards since 1974, I felt so helpless. I kept hearing, "It is all in your head, Thea." By now, I wished they would certify my "insanity." When we went for walks, I was the only patient who was totally exhausted, and at times I even collapsed. The truly mentally ill patients could walk, talk, watch TV, while I could hardly move most of the time. This was very hard for me to accept. It made no sense.

In 1986, I was in and out of the hospital for eight months with no improvement at all. This was a bitter reminder of the early 70s. At times, some of the hospital staff made hurtful remarks regarding my condition. They just could not experience the nightmare I was enduring. How could they?

Finally, after eight months, I was asked to leave the mental ward. The medical staff dared to blame me for their incapacity to diagnose my condition properly. They dropped their efforts to help me recover. And during my entire time of being hospitalized, the doctors, to my knowledge:

Never once was properly diagnosed with seizure disorder.
Never once took a simple viral panel.
Never did a toxicity test.
Never even had a neurologist examine me, even though my records showed that I had been hospitalized for two weeks after suffering a severe concussion in 1984, which resulted in major inner ear damage.*
Never once did a simple hypoglycemia test.
Never tested for Candida.
Did not ask for a professional second opinion.
Never took x-rays, even though I was in physical therapy due to severe neck and shoulder pain.

*Even though I had a seizure disorder for 25 years, during my eight-month hospital stay I was never given any seizure test or medication. At times when I did have a seizure, my roommate called for medical help, almost in hysterics, and was told not to worry. "Just let her shake, she will stop shaking." How can anyone in this day and age do this to a human being? Is it plain ignorance? I was taken to this hospital with a seizure disorder, which I have had since age 20. I felt the seizures coming on—reality left me, my body convulsed and afterward I am a zombie. It really hurts me, to this day, that no staff member would even believe I had a seizure and seeing my roommate, scared and with tears in her eyes, telling me after it was over, "Thea, I asked for help. Really I did." But **nobody** came. She told me that not only my body, but also my bed shook really badly. She feared that I would die. It is well-documented that a large number of CFIDS patients have seizure disorders.

At that time, CFIDS was in the media because of the Lake Tahoe outbreak. So why was I not checked for CFIDS? I had all the symptoms.

My illness and the attitude of the medical establishment diminished me mentally, emotionally, and financially. I lost my sense of self-worth, my dignity, and at times hope and my trust in some people.

I then was released from this mental ward in November of 1985 directly to a "half-way house" in Santa Barbara. I soon found that I did not even have the physical strength to perform the duties that all patients were required to perform. My doctor in charge (founder of the half-way house) tried to hospitalize me again and referred me to the mental ward in the same hospital where I had just been rejected. I was refused admission and instead admitted to a regular ward with a twenty-four-hour nurse. Once again, I was given six electric shock treatments.

Something dramatic and unexpected happened during my sixth electric shock treatment: cardiac arrest. The doctor called another physician in Los Angeles while the man was attending a concert and asked him if he could accept a critically ill patient. He said he would and admitted me to a Los Angeles-area hospital a few days later. I could not be hospitalized in my own town because the hospital staff there insisted that they could do nothing more for me. Perhaps they were right, but why did it take eight months to find out, leaving me with financial disaster?

I felt rejected. Now I was in a new town with a new doctor, and my family was 100 miles away.

My Special Friend Jackie: A Most Wonderful and Heartfelt Memory Forever

I tried to get used to this new hospital. It was always scary to change hospitals, as this entailed meeting new doctors and new patients, but I usually adjusted well. This is probably due to the fact that I love people and tend to get along well with others. In this particular hospital, I met a very special person.

I started going to regular group meetings. In our group, there was a seventy-six-year-old Jewish woman named Jackie. She absolutely hated the Germans and Germany and, of course, was aware that I had emigrated from Germany during World War II. No wonder that she directed all the anger that she had repressed for so many years directly onto me.

I felt great sympathy for her, because she had endured so much during the war. She said a German soldier had killed her precious child as she ran for safety. She had then spent the entire winter living in a hole she had dug in the forest, and she had nearly starved to death. Her husband had been killed during the war. How sad. I could not help but feel for her the terrible losses and the horror war brought to her.

In group therapy, Jackie directed her most hateful remarks at me. What made everything worse was that the group counselor would take her side against me. One evening quite soon after, just following the conclusion of the group therapy, I waited outside the room for the counselor, because I wanted to ask him why he would take Jackie's side and criticize me during the sessions. When I asked him, he appeared stunned, like he did not have any idea that he had taken part in persecuting me, like Jackie did. He said, "Thea, I really did not realize what I have been doing. You are right." To my surprise, he apologized for his behavior to the entire group during the next group session. He, too, had painful memories from the war and, like Jackie, was also Jewish. I broke down and cried, "Can't you understand, I was just a little child of three when the war broke out, I had nothing to do with the war or what happened to you. The war scarred me terribly, too."

Finally, during another group session in which Jackie attacked me with hateful remarks, I wanted to walk out. But something stopped me and told me that the problem would not be solved by hating this woman. So I decided to wait for her in the hallway after the group therapy ended. I saw Jackie heading for her room and walked up to her and touched her on the shoulder. As I looked into her watery eyes, I said ," Jackie, I love you, I care for you, and I need you." We both began to cry.

We hugged each other, and she invited me to come to the cafeteria with her. Happily, and with tears pouring out of my eyes, I agreed. The entire hospital could not believe the turnaround in Jackie's life from then on. She no longer spent hour after hour staring out the window, absorbed by memories of pain and death. She began eating in the cafeteria, rather than alone in her room, and she started to participate in occupational therapy. Many people, including the staff, were so touched that they cried. Even my doctor had tears in his eyes. Jackie and I became close friends. We ate together, walked together, and shared some very personal memories. After this touching experience, she was soon released to go home. I will certainly never forget Jackie, one of the truly special people I have known in my life. Wherever you are, dear Jackie, I love you very much and hope you are doing well.

Having spent so many years around the genuinely mentally ill, I can tell you that most of them live in a world all their own. In my heart, I hold very warm feelings toward them. These are very special people. Very special. There is a reason and meaning for everything. Perhaps my path had to cross this world for a higher reason. One day I will know.

I kept going on with life, wondering at times what had become of me. It is best not to wonder or analyze, because nothing really makes sense. It is best not to look back, to just follow that road, that wandering and difficult road, the road to recovery.

My dear daughter Ingrid and her wonderful husband Steve and my sister Anneliese somehow found the inner strength to stay with me and to visit me wherever I was staying. Without their love, I am certain that I would not have survived. They even had me stay at their house for a period during which I was basically bedridden. Their home was small, but they made me feel very welcome, loved, and well cared for.

My sweet little grandchildren wanted me to read bedtime stories to them, but I did not have the strength or mental concentration to do it. I could not stand any noise, even household noise. I started to withdraw, to become more and more isolated. It was just too much to watch healthy people doing normal things. My condition did not get better.

After staying with Ingrid and her loving family for a while, I decided to rent a room. However, I soon found myself very ill again. I knew I needed medical help badly, but I could not find it anywhere. Regular hospitals would not take me, yet I could not care for myself. I now know why there are so many homeless people on the streets.

Most of the time, I felt so exhausted that I didn't have the energy to cook. Often I could not even chew my food. I would cook a pot of millet and beans and blend everything in a blender. I managed just enough to stay alive. Inevitably, I got to a point where I could not even do that any more. My body continued to feel pain all over; sleep was interrupted by heavy night sweats, neck pain, and swollen lymph glands. I felt terribly sick. Was I really insane? Was I imagining my sickness? **NO!** There was something organically wrong with me. I felt it so intensely throughout all of my body that I knew it could not be an illusion. Nobody could figure it out, but I had to remind myself that someday someone would find out what was really going on with me. I often prayed, "God help me. God help me."

One day, I felt so ill that I called my doctor and talked to him about my condition. I told him that, in addition to my physical pain, I could not even eat or sleep. He wanted to hospitalize me in the mental institution again! I couldn't believe it. I knew my new insurance would not pay for a pre-existing condition, but my doctor insisted that I be hospitalized. Once I got there, the hospital staff refused to admit me. I still do not recall how I got back home to this day.

A few hours later, I took an accidental overdose of painkillers. I just could not take the pain any longer. I didn't really want to die. Sure, the pain, the feelings of rejection, the constant feeling of just barely being alive and of lying in bed alone were probably enough to trigger a death wish in almost everyone, but not in me. I never wanted to die...I just wanted relief from my pain. After I took the first two painkillers, I felt no relief. I decided to take two more, and that's when I lost control. Apparently, this painkiller did not mix very well with the medication I was taking at the time. I called my ex-husband. Thank God, he was home. He immediately called 911. The paramedics took me to the hospital, where I was admitted.

I felt terribly guilty. When my family came to visit me, they looked so worried. I can still see Elly's watery eyes. She asked me, "Why would you do this Mama?" I could not answer her right away, but deep inside of me, I knew why this horrible accident happened. I knew I would not do it again, but all of us have our weak moments. My life was going wrong. I had no answers, I just tried to keep going on.

I learned a lot from this experience. Most of all, I realized how much my illness affected my family. From then on, I have been very careful in what I take and how much—regardless of how much pain I feel. To this day, we do not talk about this incident within the family. All I can do is hope that they understand, and deep down I know they do.

Since I had no insurance, but needed further help, I was transferred to the county hospital.

Transferred to the County Hospital

A few days after this incident, I was transferred to the county hospital emergency ward. All new patients at this institution must go through emergency psychiatric examinations before being assigned to a hospital. In this particular emergency room, where the evaluations were performed, there were only eight beds and an average of 25 to 30 patients. And now began another nightmare.

Many of the new "patients" were put to sleep with powerful tranquilizers almost immediately. If not, the first thing that was done was a strip search. Every inch of my body was examined. My dignity, privacy, and all respect for me as a human being was stripped away as fast as my clothing. I felt like a piece of meat. I was allowed no control whatsoever for the first seventy-two hours, and if I didn't do as I was told, they would inject me with heavy tranquilizers on the spot.

For the most part, the staff was very decent, with some exceptions. I still remember an incident with an incredibly sadistic nurse. One night, I had to go to the bathroom. I had a urinary tract infection at the time, which is common among CFIDS sufferers. The night-duty nurse became angry at me for some reason. I seemed to have disturbed her magazine reading. When I had to get up to go to the bathroom a second time, she warned me that if I tried it again, she would give me a shot so that I would surely not get up again for the rest of the night. I warned her that the Chief of Staff of the Psychiatric Unit was a former customer at my camera store and a friend of mine and I would turn her in if she tried to inject me. It worked, and she backed off and left me alone.

Since there weren't enough beds, I had to sleep on the hard floor most of the time, together with the mentally ill and criminally insane. It felt like being squeezed into a sardine can. Some poor souls would scream, but not for long, because the heavy medication forced on them would calm them immediately. Remember that we were locked up with nowhere to go.

One psychiatrist evaluated me briefly and determined that I was suffering from major brain damage. She wanted to transfer me to the state mental institution in Camarillo, California. That would mean a minimum of six months' confinement, cloistered with thirty to thirty-five ill women in **one large room.** I was **terrified;** I felt insulted and very angry. My overwhelming fear and lack of control about this decision was almost too much to handle. But, as I said, fortunately, the Chief of Staff was a friend, and upon learning of the psychiatrist's evaluation and prognosis, he issued strict orders that I was not to be transferred to the mental institution in Camarillo or anywhere else. Thank God, they had to listen to him, or I would have been sent off at once. The only trouble was that he was about to leave for vacation, so my ultimate fate was only suspended.

I found myself in the emergency mental ward, still suffering from an undiagnosable physical illness, which had almost destroyed me. The feelings of being locked up with often dangerous people and of being powerless and totally vulnerable and weak were incredible. I was very, very sick and was forced to sleep night after night on the floor with the psychotic and criminally insane. I prayed and prayed.

I had to wait in that "snakepit" until the Chief of Staff came back from his vacation before I could know what my fate was to be.

Finally, the Chief of Staff returned from his vacation. I was then transferred to the sixth floor of the same medical center to another unit of the mental ward and locked up. The Chief of Staff came to visit me once or twice a day, as did several other doctors who took an interest in my case. They all agreed that I certainly did not have major brain damage, but no one could tell me what I did have. However, I was very happy and relieved to not have been sent to the state mental institution. In the past, while in other mental institutions, I had been physically attacked and beaten for no reason by patients who were too ill to even know that they were doing anything wrong.

As I look back, I cannot believe how lucky I was that some very special people believed in me and in my worth as a human being. Those eleven days I had to wait for the Chief of Staff to return from his vacation were beyond any nightmare I had ever experienced. If I failed to "meet the standard" of the county hospital, I would then be transferred to the final stop: a state institution. That probably would have been the final stop for Thea Schlosser. If I were to be put in a room with thirty or so other people to live and sleep, I knew I could not take it. My entire head hurt all of the time. To be forced to live with the noise and true mental illness of thirty others in one room would certainly be the end of my life.

Please understand, I have nothing against mentally ill people. As a matter of fact, I cared for and loved each one of them. But some were dangerous; some talked to themselves; some would just sit there and stare, with no expression on their faces; some would come right off the streets, drunk and in despair; some would scream, cry, and go into hysterics; and others would simply wash their hands all day. Being in the delicate state that I was in, it was very hard for me to deal with their problems, as well as mine. I learned a lot about life in those eleven days, and in the past years since then.

Why So Cruel?

I had no choice but to adjust to the new ward, which was definitely much more bearable than the emergency psychiatric ward where I had been for the previous eleven days. There was never a moment of happiness, never a moment of peace, and I never felt safe. It is very hard to be in a mental ward and see the patients with such sad, empty expressions. But the fact that my children were alive and loved me, even if I was beyond their immediate reach and help, kept me going. My sister Anneliese, who visited me often, as well as many of my friends and family, never lost faith in me, especially my daughter Ingrid and her husband Steve.

One evening, the charge nurse suggested that I go to the "Quiet Room" and hit the pillow, since I was still angry about the doctor who said that I was brain damaged and wanted to send me to the state hospital that kept me for eleven days in the county psychiatric emergency room for no reason. This seemed like a good idea to me. Being kept under such devastating conditions for days and the heavy medication they had me on did not allow me to release any of my feelings.

We went to the **"Quiet Room,"** and I began to hit the pillow. It felt GREAT! It helped me start to release some of the rage that I had kept deep inside me for so long. Suddenly, the charge nurse stopped me from hitting the pillow. I wondered why, but all she said was, "No more Thea, I have to go on with my medication rounds now." I begged her, "No! We cannot stop now. Please, I am just beginning to feel better." I had just been transferred from spending eleven days in the "snakepit," and I was still trying to come to terms with that outrage. Equally mortifying was the fact that I had been declared "brain damaged." I had just been given something that helped me, and it was taken away from me. Why? I could not understand that. "Please, no," I said again. How could I possibly stop hitting the pillow after just a few minutes? That was more than I could handle. The charge nurse stopped me anyway. I then began to shake and tremble. I asked her for medication. As she refused, my rage made me grab and shove a small table. Instantly, four nurses jumped at me and dragged me to a "special" room, where I was tied down to a bed.

First, I was encouraged to hit the pillow, and then it was abruptly taken away from me. Now, because I was angry about that, I was tied to a bed, treated the same way as the most dangerous cases in that hospital. The worst part was that I have **"restless leg" syndrome,**

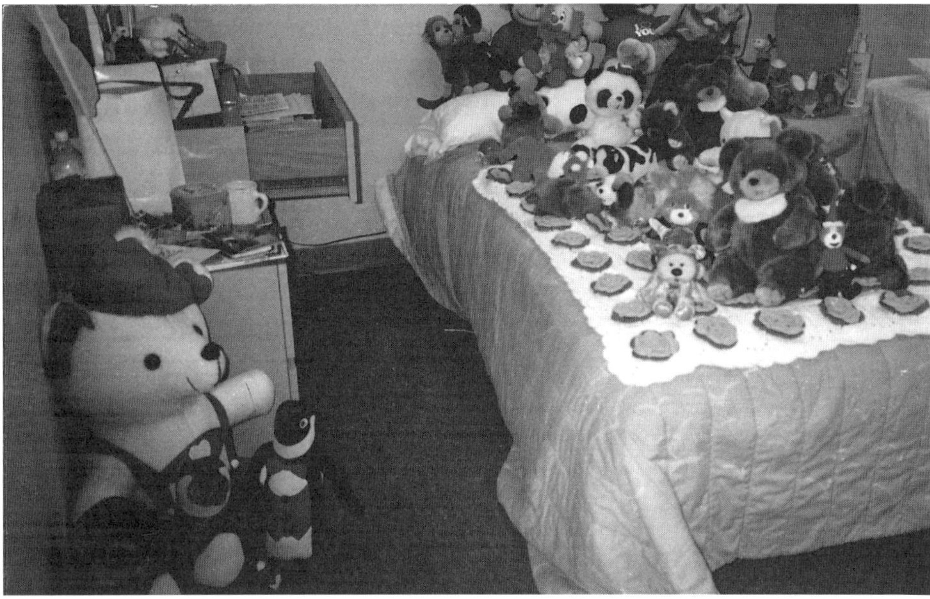

Because I missed my family and friends so much while staying at the half-way house, I started to collect stuffed animals and made them my temporary family.

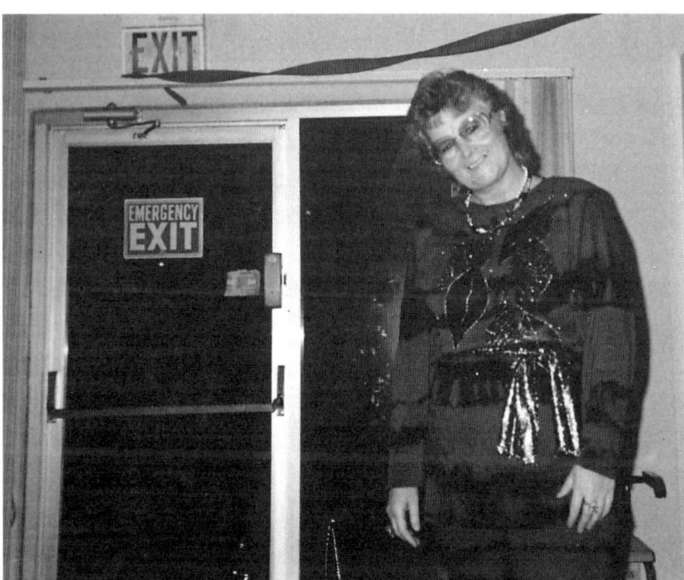

New Year's 1987 in the half-way house. With all the antidepressant medication I was taking, I gained fifty-five pounds. Although the antidepressants did not work, I kept smiling, hoping that some day soon I would know what was wrong with me.

common to Chronic Fatigue Syndrome patients, and now I could not even move my legs, not even an inch. Nothing helped to relieve the overwhelming grief I felt from being tied up like an animal almost until dawn the next day. Every second felt like ten hours. Crying was my only source of relief. Why so cruel? I asked myself. I did not harm anybody! Kicking the table slightly was also due to total exhaustion and fear—fear of the state hospital, some nurses and patients, and eleven days in a room with 25 to 30 patients. Day and night felt the same—the lights never went out; the screaming of other patients did not stop; it was madness; it was worse than World War II. The nurse should have understood that I was at my end. Then again, they see patients all the time, and I was just another one.

I do not think that I can ever forget this inhuman act. I thought about all those **poor souls,** who regularly, for their safety, must be tied down. I also think about all of the people who were tied down for no reason at all. I really do not want to judge anyone, but I did feel that some of the staff actually did **enjoy** doing those things **to the patients. It gave them power. While writing this section, the memories were so painful, so inhumane, so degrading, so indescribable, that I had to stop writing for two weeks.**

Two days after this humiliating incident, I "graduated" from the hospital to a half-way house. This house was also connected with county facilities for the mentally ill. After six more weeks on the third floor, under lock-up conditions, and then two more transfers to other facilities, the decision was made to transfer me into a "half-way house" again. During this period, I actually enrolled in a class at Los Angeles City College. I wanted to become a counselor for alcoholics and drug addicts. Unfortunately, I could not finish it. I was too ill and exhausted, but I tried anyway. I just kept looking for ways to get back into life. I was very disappointed.

According to the half-way house rules, I had to share twenty hours of cooking, cleaning, and gardening with the twenty other residents. I also had to take care of my own home, rented from the city. I had neither the physical strength nor the mental clarity to perform the required work.

After sharing a room with a woman for four months, I learned that she was a convicted murderess who had killed her own child. I remember vomiting when I found out. After five months, I was told that I was going to be put through a complete physical check-up back at the county hospital again. By now, some of the doctors and staff members in the half-way house had observed me long enough to start thinking that my problem could be physical and not mental. They finally realized that I was in the wrong part of the medical system. They could no longer justify my stay in a county-operated mental facility, because there was nothing mentally wrong with me. For the most part, I was optimistic, friendly, and willing to help, although I felt very ill and exhausted. It was a good-news, bad-news situation, and I became even more fearful. I was being informed that I was not even qualified for the mentally ill rehabilitation program. Where could I go if I was not diagnosed with something? I was too ill to care for myself.

The people at the county facility were good people. But they received more than three hundred and seventy-five calls every day requesting space in the half-way house for the mentally ill who *could* do the required physical work. They didn't want to let me go, but they had no choice.

Two days later I went out to a neighborhood health food store and just happened to pick up a health magazine. I saw an advertisement in a magazine that was to **SAVE MY LIFE.**

FINALLY, CORRECTLY DIAGNOSED!

The ad featured a questionnaire that asked questions like:

Do you have night sweats?

Do you have headaches?

Are you fatigued all of the time?

Do you have severe muscle pain?

Do you have swollen glands?

Do the doctors tell you that "it is all in your head?"

I literally could not believe what my eyes were reading. I read the questions again. Yes! They all applied! The ad talked about a new disease called **"Chronic Fatigue and Immune Dysfunction."** I had never heard of anything like it before. Who had put such an ad in this magazine? A medical clinic in Tijuana, Mexico. Was this a joke? Thank God that it was not.

The name and diagnosis sounded interesting, and it felt that this might be the answer to what was going on with me. I had nothing to lose, so I telephoned the clinic. Within forty-eight hours, I arrived at the clinic in Mexico, thanks to my ex-husband Karl, who picked me up at the half-way house and drove me there—no questions asked. He also handed me enough cash so I could survive.

I could always depend on Karl. Not only did he always pay his alimony on time, but he also helped me out financially. This goes to show that even when people divorce, they can still be human to each other. I am eternally grateful to Karl for many of the sacrifices he made for the children and me. This one probably saved my life.

When I arrived at the clinic, I was very, very sick. I had an extremely severe case of systemic Candida. I had it vaginally and rectally, and it was even *growing on my skin.* I had fungus growing on my nails, ears, and on my tongue. I was almost being consumed by yeast. The clinic doctors conducted several tests and confirmed with certainty that I was suffering from Chronic Fatigue and Immune Dysfunction. My symptoms included severe Fibromyalgia, which is like a severe form of arthritis affecting most parts of the body, and massive, near fatal, Candida, along with severe hypoglycemia, hypothyroidism, and anemia. I was glad that I had a diagnosis, but, sadly, I had to leave the American medical system to get it.

The emotions that overcame me were *indescribable.* My unknown, phantom, ruthless, vile disease, the stealer of my life for so many years, *was physical* and ***it had a name!*** "Chronic Fatigue and Immune Dysfunction." "Chronic Fatigue Syndrome." "Yuppie Flu." Along with tidy little acronyms such as "CFIDS" and "CFS." It had acquired millions of victims, many of whom were suffering in silence and ignorance, like I had been.

If someone were to tell you that you suffered from an incurable disease, you would probably become sad and depressed. But not me. I felt like **I was the happiest sick person on Earth!** It was now

1989, and I had been victimized by this disease since 1970. I had just survived the last five years of my life being processed and violated by hospitals, more than a few sadists, and too many mental institutions. Now my disease had finally been given a name. Through **renewed hope,** I had been **given back my life.** What was left of it.

At first, all I could think about was how I was going to recover. I thought that Chronic Fatigue would be easy to treat once it had been diagnosed. I hoped that I could get back to my family and work soon. To my surprise, this was not the case. Actually, the CFIDS patients I saw at the clinic in Mexico looked worse than any other patients I had ever seen. They even looked worse than the patients who had cancer. Cancer patients were at least able to shop, watch television, and put on make-up. The CFIDS patients looked pale, acted confused and depressed at times, and rested in their beds more than anyone else at the clinic. I, of course, was one of them.

Climbing the Mountain

As I commit these memories and tribulations to paper, and virtually every day of my life, **I wonder how many hundreds or thousands of others** have had to **go through similar tragedies?** How many thousands of others have been **confined to mental wards,** been made to **strip naked, been injected with tranquilizers, been given electric shock treatments,** and continue to **be utterly and totally degraded by this horrible disease?** The fear that there may be someone out there just like me who might be reached and saved from ignorant health care practitioners keeps me writing a diary.

The road back to good health is never an easy one when dealing with a catastrophic illness. Just getting **the proper diagnosis,** under the best of conditions and circumstances, is a chance situation. Your blood test may come back "relatively" normal, the doctors begin to flow past you in an almost endless stream, and still no diagnosis. Thankfully, more and more doctors, but not nearly enough, are now aware of CFIDS, even if they are not particularly well-versed in its treatment, minimal as it may be.

Little did I realize that many, many hurdles lay immediately before me, some even worse than what I had already experienced. The staff members at the clinic in Mexico were fantastic. My assigned doctor was a dedicated physician.

I was put on an intravenous mixture containing Vitamin C, along with many minerals. I was given a Candida fighter, Dioxclor; an amino acid, L-Taurine; and an anti-viral drug, Isoprinosine. I was also given regular coffee enemas. After three weeks, I was able to go home!

Although the immediate treatment was successful, six months later, the long, cold, gray hand of illness grabbed me once again. I had such unbearable headaches that I was bedridden for weeks. I finally called my daughter Ingrid and asked her to come over right away. After seeing my condition, she called the clinic in Mexico. The doctor urged her to bring me to back right away.

Karl and Ingrid immediately took me down to Tijuana. We arrived on a Saturday at 10:00 p.m. We were exhausted. Karl and Ingrid drove back to Santa Barbara that same night. They knew I was in good hands.

The staff quickly went to work to assess my condition. Their diagnosis: severe viral encephalitis.

At times I had three to six major seizures a day, which lasted three weeks. After the three weeks the seizures were less and less frequent. If I had not been under such competent care, the results could have been fatal. Just eight months earlier, my American physicians were telling me that there was nothing physically wrong with me. **"Thea, it's all in your head,"** they said. There were many, many nights when sleep eluded me entirely. I was clearly fighting for my life. My body knew it, and so did my mind.

This time, I had to spend three months in the clinic. The financial burden was huge. Since I had very little or no insurance, Ingrid and Steve mortgaged their home to partially pay for my hospitalization. Karl also helped me financially.

I was somehow able to rally myself again. I was termed barely well enough to be able to leave the hospital and return to Santa Barbara, where I managed to find a room for rent in a home. The lady of the household took care of me much of the time. Most disturbingly, the pain in my neck, which resulted from old injuries, had now become so intense that I considered it an ugly, equal twin

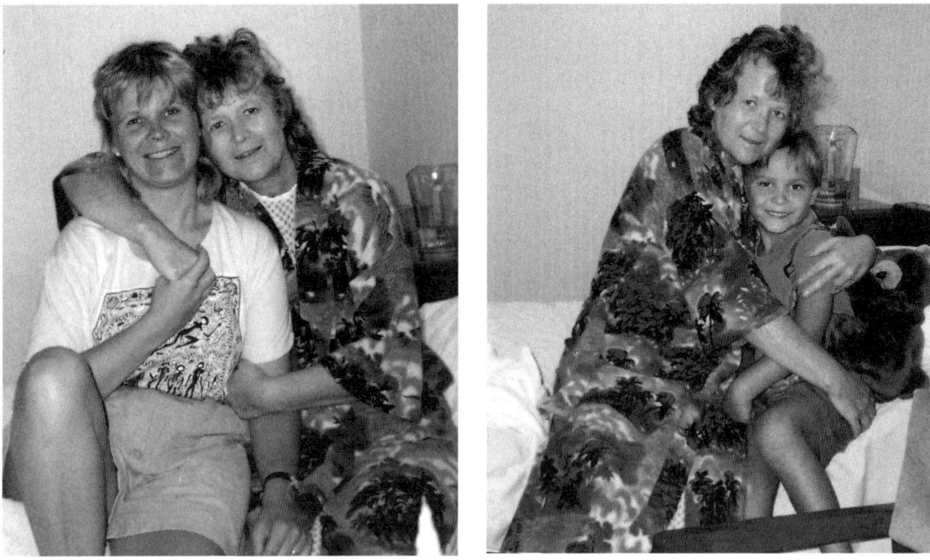

Ingrid visited me wherever I was. Here we are in Mexico, where I was recuperating from encephalitis.

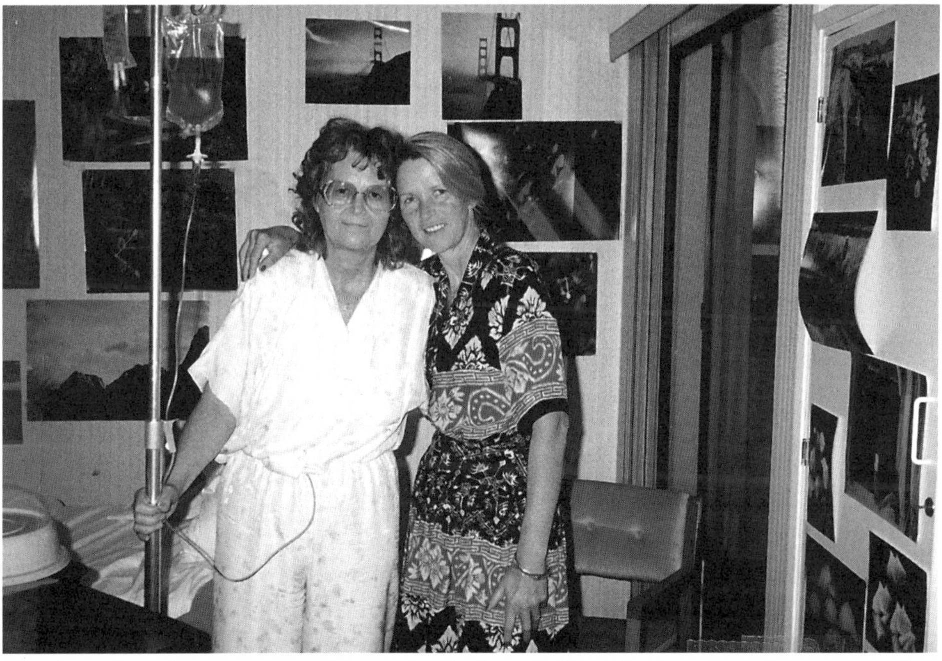

My sister Anneliese came to visit me in the hospital in Mexico where I was recovering from encephalitis. As you can see, I decorated my room with pictures that I had taken in order to try to forget how ill I was and concentrate on life's beauty.

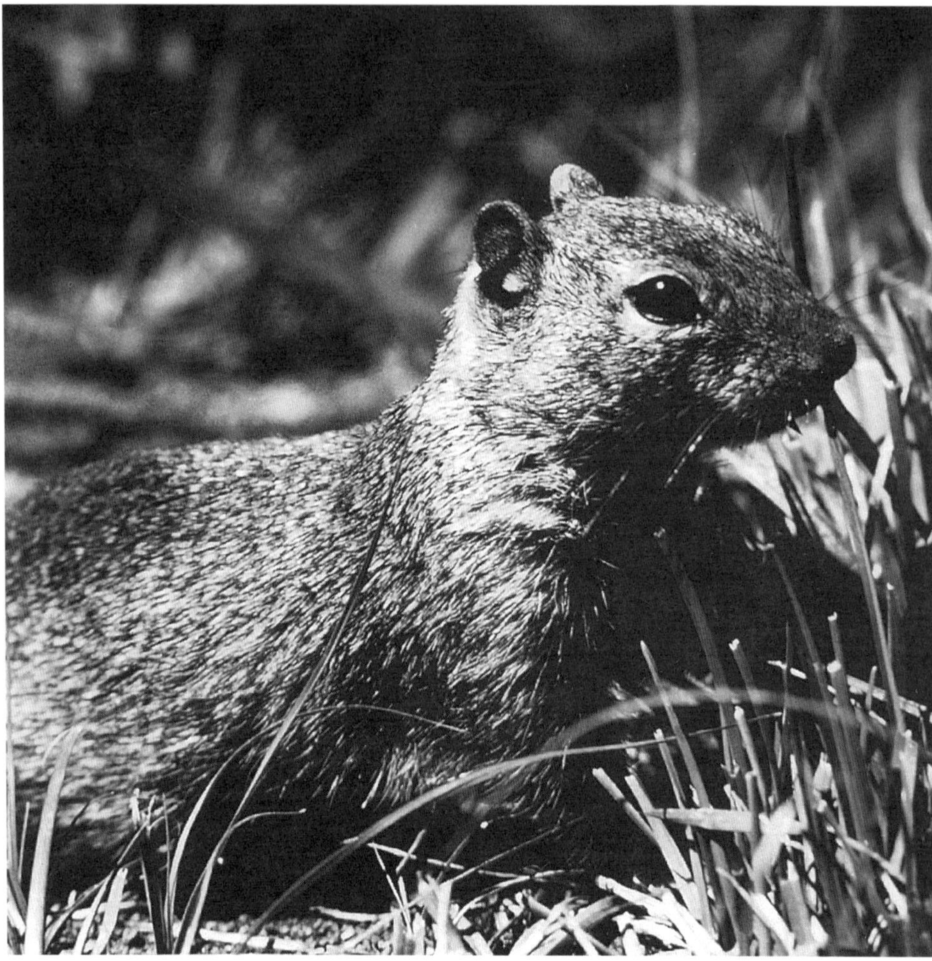

Photo by Thea.

of my Chronic Fatigue Syndrome. At this point I really would like to say that we in America have some of the finest medical doctors and scientists, but their training is in mainstream medical treatment. It would be nice if our fine doctors in the USA would update their medical treatment and be more open-minded to alternative treatments.

In June of 1990, I was well enough to be discharged from the clinic. I was known as their "miracle patient." Not only did I recover from the common CFIDS viruses such as CMV, EBV, Herpes I and VI, and Candida, but I also overcame the encephalitis. Wonderful medical care, love, and God gave me a new start.

A New Start

By January 17, 1993, I had my own apartment again. After eight years in houses and mental wards, I finally had my own "home" again. First, I had feelings of fear and of being overwhelmed. *Sensory overload!* But those feelings changed rather quickly into a feeling of freedom. I had no one to answer to. I had my own space. **And I loved it!**

The most difficult task for me was shopping. What a terrible obstacle for me. Luckily, Ingrid and Steve were nearby to help me once again. At this time, I founded *The Chronic Fatigue and Immune Dysfunction Media Awareness Association.* CFIDS was still my constant companion, sharing equal time with my ever-worsening neck pain, which was a disaster in itself by this time. I began to seek chiropractic help for it. Nothing helped. In July of 1993, I collapsed from the sheer exhaustion of having to fight off the pain virtually twenty-four hours a day, along with dealing with CFIDS.

Clinic in Tijuana

Shortly after I collapsed from the pain and exhaustion, it was clear that I would have to return to the hospital in Mexico. Once there, I was told that my body was hosting multiple infections, including Candida, Herpes, and CVM (Herpes IV). I was so ill that I hadn't actually realized how sick I was. By the time I was hospitalized, I didn't care where I was anymore.

At this point, I was told that I would need to have neck surgery due to the fact that I had several extra cervical ribs coming off the vertebrae in my neck. I decided to have the surgery in Mexico, since I was already there, and the medical team wanted to build up my immune system first. To this day, I hardly remember going through the surgical procedure at all. First, I was told, the surgery took five hours.

DISCHARGE SUMMARY

NAME: THEA SCHLOSSER

FILE: 2894

ADMISSION DATE: November 20-1989

DISCHARGE DATE: December 11-1989

DIAGNOSIS: Chronic Fatigue Syndrome
Hypothyroidism
Generalized Seizures (epilepsy)
Chronic Estrogen Intake
Chronic Colitis
Enlarged Uterus/Probable Endometriosis

HISTORY OF PRESENT ILLNESS: This is a 52 year old lady; who refers she initiated having health problems since 25 years ago consistent with malaise, fatigue and emotional depression. Five years ago her condition worsened so since then she has not been able to work. She has frequent headaches, forgets simple things easily, she has generalized muscle and joint aches, night sweats, severe abdominal pains, diarrhea and constipation alterned no blood on stools. She will also present on a monthly cycle severe pelvic pain accompanied by malaise and occasionally fever. Four weeks ago she presented her last generalized seizure she was diagnosed with epilepsy a year ago presently under control with Dilantin 300 mg and Tegretol, she occasionally will require Valium. At the present time she is having general malaise, fatigue which is severe to the point where she cannot get out of bed. She presents pelvic pain, vaginal discharge and constipation. She is not able to eat so she has lost around 15 pounds in about 2 weeks.

PAST MEDICAL HISTORY: She had the usual childhood illnesses; she was diagnosed with epilepsy a year ago presently under control with Dilantin, Tegretol and Valium. She suffers from some kind of Immune-depression since approximately 25 years ago because since this time she has presented frequent infections and multiple antibiotic treatments have been recommended. She suffers from a chronic pelvic inflamation since about a year ago multiple treatments she has received without benefit she has several vaginal cultures positive for different bacteria.

1989. Finally, correctly diagnosed. This is my discharge summary from the clinic in Mexico.

Chronic constipation is a problem though she tries to stay on a healthy diet. Due to her diversity of symptoms and emotional stress, no definite diagnosis had been made and she was in a mental institution for about a year receiving electric shock and multiple mood elevators.

FAMILY HISTORY

Her father died of cancer and her mother suffered from high blood pressure and thyroid disease she committed suicide at 46. Thea has 2 healthy children.

SOCIAL HISTORY

Thea is a photographer and was involved in business up until 5 years ago with good success. She does not drink alcohol nor smoke. She does not take any drugs. She is presently receiving Dilantin 300 mg and occasionally will take 2.5 mg of Diazepam for her epilepsy. She does take a daily Synthroid supplement and Premarin.

HOSPITAL COURSE: Thea remained hospitalized with us for about 20 days, she tolerated everything fairly well; she did have a severe attack of colitis and her pelvic problem flared up. She received treatment with antibiotics, antivirals, her seizure medication was continued so as thyroid which was decreased since she was taking too much. Her general condition during her stay went down for a few days when she was not able to get out of bed. Vaginal cultures showed infection with Candida, Gardnerella Vaginalis, and Staphylococcus aureus, Viral levels to Herpes S, Epstein Barr and Cytomegalovirus very abnormal. Liver profile very abnormal since about 3 months ago almost consistent with hepatitis; for this reason Dilantin was decreased for several days until liver was almost normal. Pelvic ultrasound demonstrates an enlarged uterus and atrophied ovaries, the patient takes Premarin since 30 years of age. Chest xrays were normal. Pap smear showed moderate to severe inflamation. At the time of discharge Thea was feeling better she was able to take care of herself and of course was more energetic. She was pending the proposition of the gynecologist to have an hysterectomy due to the multiple problems her enlarged uterus is producing all probably secondary to chronic estrogen intake.

PHYSICAL EXAMINATION: Mostly normal except for a yellowish skin color, painful colon, enlarged uterus and vaginal atrophy.

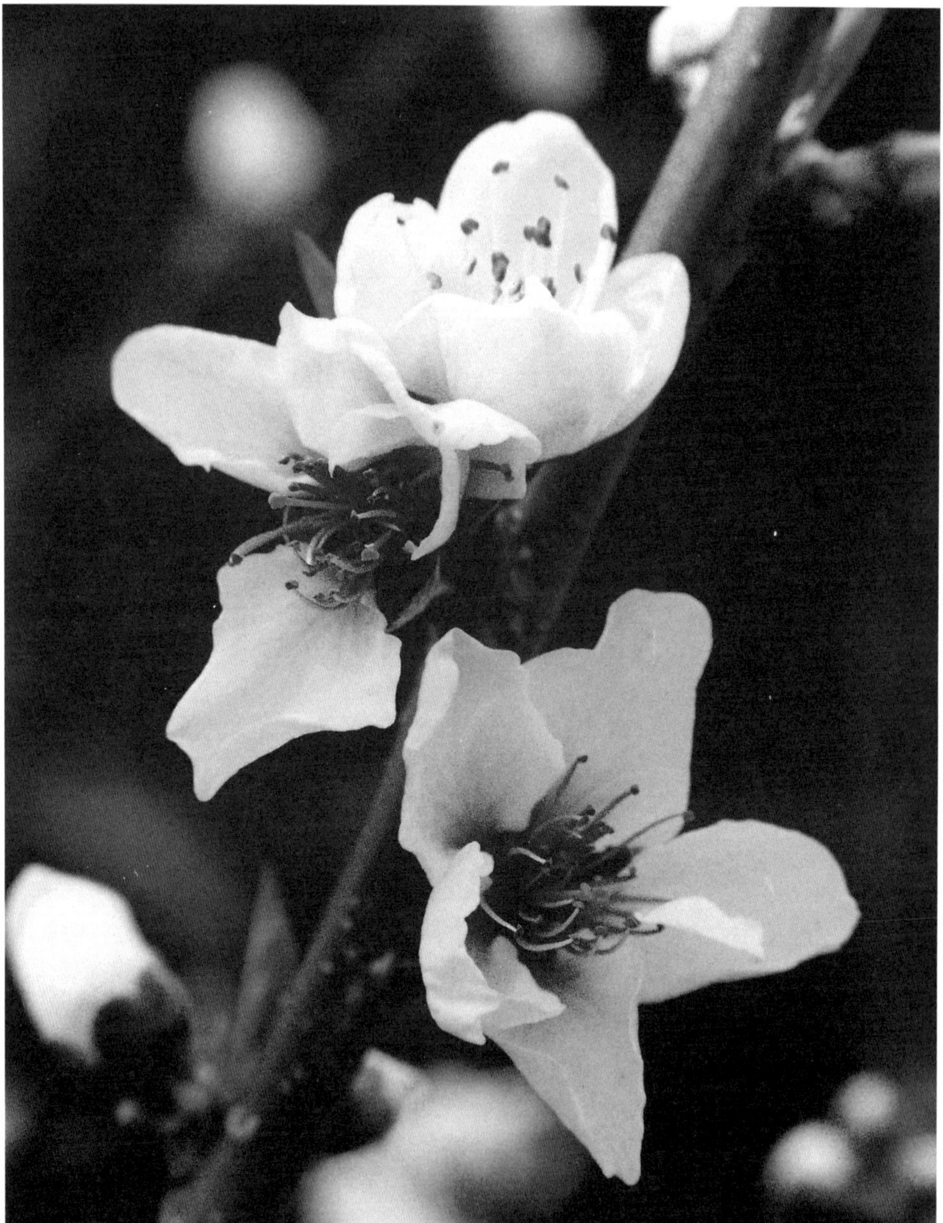

Photo by Thea. This peach blossom reminds me of "life's cycle," as it will one day become a delicious peach. Every day of our lives is a new start. What we do with it is completely up to us.

I could not move one inch. I was completely immobilized. There was also a communication barrier, as I did not speak Spanish and most of the staff did not speak English. Make no mistake, everyone was very pleasant to me, and the quality of care was very good, but there were these obstacles to deal with that patients in American hospitals don't encounter. I will never, ever forget the graciousness and kindness that I received from the people in Mexico. Both in and out of the hospital.

After two weeks of recovery from the surgery, I was driven back home to Santa Barbara by a friend. This was decidedly a mistake on my part, because every bump in the road and intersection stops and starts were painful on my still immobilized neck. In any case, I was going home, and I was happy!

As unbelievable as this may sound, my neck condition actually worsened. The extra vertebrae rib surgery was not enough. The x-rays showed other problems. My spinal cord measured a compression level of three, four, and five, with bone spurs growing. Painkillers did virtually nothing. I could not sleep, I lost weight, and I was in bed most of the time. Six weeks later, I had to have another neck surgery.

I flew to Mexico. This time, they had to fuse the vertebrae in order to stabilize my neck. The doctors huddled, and the prevailing wisdom was that pieces of bone from my hip should be harvested and placed between the troublesome vertebrae in my neck. They were thoughtful enough to inquire whether I might prefer some bone pieces taken from a cadaver. I declined. The thought of bone from a dead body inside of me gave me the chills.

The surgery lasted more than five hours, almost identical in time to the first. Two days after the procedure, I developed a serious fever and shortness of breath. The doctors ordered x-rays and confirmed that there was water in my lungs, I had pleurisy, and my diaphragm was pushed up against one of my lungs because of a nerve that was injured during surgery. I was in critical condition for two days. It was scary, but with faith in the Almighty, we can do almost anything.

After a two-week hospital stay, I finally flew back home to Santa Barbara. To my disappointment and despair, the neck pain remained. Once again, I sought help through chiropractic treatment. Again, with marginal, temporary results. I also received physical therapy twice a week, but to little avail. My chiropractor suggested that I see a friend of his who is a distinguished neurosurgeon. By this time, I had acquired insurance, so I went to see him. I was immediately put through yet another battery of tests. The results confirmed severe cervical compression. Worse yet, the tests demonstrated that the surgical fusion had actually *disintegrated* and the vertebrae were no longer being held together. It was clear that yet another surgery was mandatory. The old cliché, "the third time's the charm" was of little consolation to me. Unfortunately, there really wasn't much to discuss. The surgery had to be performed. So, for the third time in eight months, I underwent neck surgery. The hospital was not in Mexico this time, but an hour-and-a-half south of Santa Barbara, just north of Los Angeles. The procedure was set for four-and-a-half hours, if all went well. Time slipped away, as it always does, and I woke up with my neck immobilized and trussed. I remained in the hospital for five days, and then Ingrid drove me home. As always, the pain in my neck was still there.

I began to sink into what is commonly referred to as "post-surgical" depression. The pain had not abated in the least from the operation. It became quite clear that no one had been able to figure out what was causing my neck pain. I was in constant pain. And I was sick with Chronic Fatigue Syndrome.

Mexico Again: This Time for Neck Surgery

My friend and physician, Professor Wolfram Kühnau, came up from Mexico to visit me at my small apartment in Santa Barbara. When he saw my condition, he was very concerned. Within minutes, he announced that I was going to get into his car and be driven back to Mexico for proper rest and, hopefully, recuperation. He felt that I should enter the hospital, so I did. All I knew was that I wanted to live. I took a moment to leave a message on my answering machine saying that I would be back in a week or two, sometime in the middle of September. I did not return until November 8, 1993.

I was not in good condition. When I arrived at the clinic, I was suffering from a severe sinus infection and a raging case of Candida. This debilitating infection, so common in people with Chronic Fatigue, is often very difficult to bring under control. I was also having seizures again. Being hospitalized is never easy, I would know probably as well as anyone, but I must say that the staff and facilities were as good as I've ever experienced. I had actually wanted to visit Mexico again, just not as a patient. But as a patient it was. Angiograms and x-rays had to be done, but I was too sick to tolerate the procedures for weeks to come. Sleeping at night wasn't possible. That is one of the most common problems with Chronic Fatigue Syndrome patients; no matter how tired you get, you can still have trouble sleeping. On top of all of this, my neck pain was so intense that it literally obliterated what little physical strength I had. When CFS would flare up with a viral outbreak, be it Herpes or Epstein-Barr, the pain in my neck seemed ten times worse. The glands in my neck would swell to a ridiculous size, and every muscle in my body would seem to burn as if on fire. This condition, known as Fibromyalgia, is extremely painful. Unfortunately, it was accompanied by the usual symptoms of CFIDS.

The doctors did their best. I was given antibiotics to knock down the multiple bacterial infections. Unfortunately, antibiotics also kill off the good bacteria in your body, which worsened my Candida. And to top it all off, I was told that I needed another neck surgery, but there was no way that could occur until my immune system was built up again.

I was given anti-fungal medication for the Candida. For the viral infections, such as Herpes, I was given Zovirax. This was a truly vicious cycle, and no matter how much nutritional support I was given, the amount of medication was taking a heavy toll on my body. I was essentially playing a waiting game with what had passed for a "life" for so many years. I was alone. I was physically and emotionally depleted. The word despair no longer applied to me. I was beyond it. And yet I persevered.

Because my veins collapse easily, the doctors had to perform minor surgery on my chest in order to put a tube in my main artery. This would enable the hospital to treat me intravenously or take blood, without the added strain of trying to find a usable vein.

I spent another four months of my life in the hospital, essentially bedridden. Praying helped. And certainly my family helped to support me, as did the wonderful staff. During many of the days that went by, like so many ants in a trail, I would do my best to write this story down. I wrote in longhand, which was barely legible to others, but to me, it represented the beginnings of great hope that my ordeal could somehow be turned into a positive experience for myself and for others. It also gave me a sense of self-worth as a human being. I felt that I had something of value to give to others. Something meaningful. A book was still a dream. A dream that felt too far away to reach, but there was a little flame glowing somewhere inside of me that one day *Beyond The Dark Cloud* would come to be.

Sundays seemed to be the hardest on me. It seemed that almost everyone else was having fun and enjoying life. I missed my family more than I can adequately express with words. I would often place their faxes, letters, cards, and photos up on the wall, but then it became too painful for me to even look at them, and down they would come. We get an empty feeling when we are not able to do things for others, because we are so often hospitalized. When I felt emotionally better again, I would retrieve the pictures and put them back up. It was a strange, bittersweet reminder, which provided me great warmth at one moment, but could quickly degenerate into near grief the next.

The medical care at the clinic was genuinely advanced. Not necessarily with respect to high-tech gadgetry, but advanced in the sense that they employ many natural methods and techniques for healing that allow for the use of traditional pharmaceuticals to be minimized whenever possible. Some of the extraordinary and extremely beneficial therapies I have received include live cells, Rife machine, ozone, and chelation therapy. All of these technologies should be readily available in the United States. Tragically, that is not the case. I do feel that we in America are taking too much medicine and not taking advantage of the many natural and alternative treatments used in other countries.

This time, the surgery was a success, to a point. The fusion held, but the pain never left. I desperately looked for answers. Naturally, I was disappointed. So were the doctors. Someone suggested that I see a certain **osteopathic physician.** This was a turning point on my way to recovery. I finally started to get more and more relief from head, neck and shoulder pain. I experienced less headaches and dizziness, as well as increased energy.

Apparently, most of my head and neck problems resulted from the concussion I suffered in 1984, along with the swimming pool injury I sustained in Austria when I was fourteen.

I was hopeful to finally have an answer for my pain. I could not have gone on much longer. I feel that anyone suffering from eye, neck, or headache pain should see a good osteopathic doctor. It changed my life for the better.

It really takes a long time to get better, and it is very costly, but I look forward to the time when I can do things again and have more energy. I especially look forward to being with my family and friends more often. One day, I will also be able to enjoy photography and going to the theater and swimming again.

Conclusion and Being Able to Enjoy Life Again

In the past pages, I did not write a lot about good experiences in my life, because I wanted to zero in on when I got ill, how I endured, and the recovery process. I did not want it to be a biography alone. I tried to share with you the obstacles that I had to overcome. Now that I feel better, I appreciate life more, because my senses are more alive. My hopes for a better future are not only dreams; they are the reality.

I am able to connect with my family better.

Recovering from CFIDS feels more and more like reaching the top of the highest mountain on a winding and, at times, invisible road.

I can already have company for a few days. I call my daughters and their families more frequently. Life is coming back to me, perhaps not fast enough, or perhaps I am a little impatient, but what a great feeling to feel that **dark** cloud *lifting.*

Regardless of how dark the cloud, or how painful the road to recovery is, remember always that we are all capable of feeling that **heavy cloud lift,** feeling and seeing the **gracious warm rays of the sun again. Despair** can change to **hope.** This I know, and this you may feel one day, if you're not feeling it already. Then, other people's **ignorance** will not hurt so much any more. The feeling of being **"brain dead"** might soon only be an infrequent **bad dream.** We can turn the **rejections** of the past into **spiritual growth** and remember those people who are in need with more understanding. **Anger** and **hurt** can be **replaced** with **love for yourself and love for others.**

I wish I could share with you that I am totally recovered, but the sad truth is I am not. The good news is that I am feeling much better now, and for that I am very grateful.

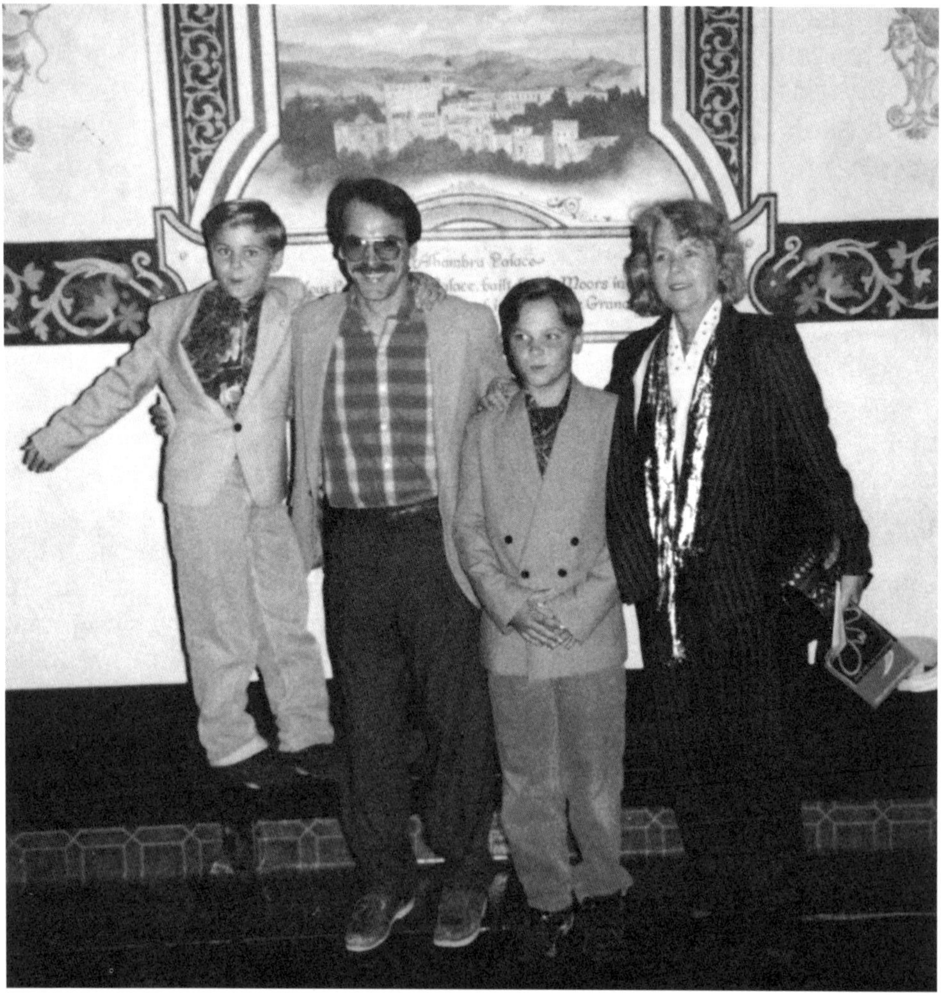

It felt great to go to a musical in Santa Barbara with my son-in-law Steve and my two grandchildren.

We are not asking for nor want sympathy; sympathy is only another form of insult. What we do need is compassion and understanding.

From the many letters and phone calls that I receive, I feel the tremendous courage from each CFIDS survivor. The search for healing and relief from CFIDS is, at times, overwhelming. Too many CFIDS survivors are still ignored or labeled as lazy, mentally ill, or hypochondriacs to this day! Rejected from mainstream society. Is it not sad? A better word for it is **CRUEL.**

We, as a society, need to recognize that CFIDS is an **illness** and deal with it in any way that we can. It is my wish that **soon** the "dark cloud" lift for all of us.

Please notice the photo of the dark cloud that I took for the front cover of this book. If you look closely, you will see that the sun is shining through. This symbol was meant for all of us—

"Beyond The Dark Cloud."

TO THE READER

As you may know, I started to write *Beyond The Dark Cloud* in 1990. The previous pages of my biography have ended on a positive note. For this reason, it may confuse you as you begin to read the symptoms and coping skills and may seem as if I am still very ill. The book reads this way because the symptoms and coping skills were written at a time when I was still very ill. As I have slowly improved over the years, I felt it was important to write as I felt at that time. Also, separating the biography from coping skills and symptoms makes it easier for the reader. I gave this much thought.

—Thea

Chapter Two

What is CFIDS?

Definition of CFIDS

CFIDS (Chronic Fatigue and Immune Dysfunction Syndrome) is also known as CFS (Chronic Fatigue Syndrome), CEBV (Chronic Epstein-Barr Virus), ME (Myalgic Encephalomyelitis), and "Yuppie Flu," among many other names. This complex illness is characterized by incapacitating fatigue, experienced as exhaustion and extremely poor stamina, neurological problems, and a constellation of symptoms that can resemble many disorders, including Mononucleosis, Multiple Sclerosis, Fibromyalgia, AIDS-Related Complex, Lyme Disease, Post-Polio Syndrome, and auto-immune diseases such as Lupus. All segments of the population, including children, are at risk, but women under the age of forty-five seem to be most susceptible. There seems to be more women than men afflicted with CFIDS.

What Causes CFIDS?

Research suggests that CFIDS results from a dysfunction of the immune system. The exact nature of this dysfunction is not yet well defined, but it can generally be viewed as an overactive state, which is responsible for most of the symptoms. Ironically, there is also evidence of some immune suppression in CFIDS; patients exhibit certain down-regulated signs. For example, many patients have functional deficiencies in natural killer cells, an important component of the immune system responsible for protection against viruses and cancer.

For a period of time, it was thought that the Epstein-Barr virus (EBV), which causes mononucleosis, was the cause of the syndrome. However, researchers now believe, that in most cases, EBV activation (when it exists) is a result of CFIDS complications, rather than its cause.

In a study published in the April '91 issue of *Proceedings of the National Academy of Sciences,* a team of researchers discovered evidence of a retro-virus in more than 75% of thirty-one CFIDS patients studied. They also found the same viral sequence in about one-third of twenty healthy persons exposed to PWCs (in close, but casual, non-sexual contact). None of the twenty healthy, "non-exposure" controls showed the presence of such virus-positive cells in their blood. These and other recent findings suggest that a retro-virus is associated with CFIDS and may be directly involved in causing the disease in many PWCs.

Research efforts are still directed toward identifying and isolating the fundamental agent(s) responsible for triggering immune system dysfunction in PWCs. Additionally, there are ongoing studies of abnormalities found in the immune system and co-factors (such as genetic predisposition, age, sex, prior illness, other viruses, environment, and stress) that appear to play an important role in the development and course of the illness.

How Can CFIDS Be Treated and What is the Prognosis?

No primary therapy has been proven to cure CFIDS. However, trials are underway with Ampligen, Kutapressin, and other experimental treatment methods. In addition, some symptoms can be frequently lessened by prescription drugs such as Klonopon, Prozac, Sinequan, Xanax, and Zantac. These must be carefully tailored to the need of each individual and often must be taken in unusually low dosages. Also, avoidance of environmental irritants and certain foods can sometimes relieve symptoms, and a number of PWCs claim to have benefited from nutritional and other non-conventional therapies. A significant percentage of PWCs show marked improvement over time. But many remain ill or cycle through a continuing series of remissions and relapses. The symptoms in severely affected PWCs can be devastating and result in prolonged interruption of work and family life. Some researchers believe that PWCs may also be at greater risk of developing Multiple Sclerosis or other illnesses. However, the extent to which CFIDS may be progressive or degenerative is not yet known. For additional information or treatment options and prognosis, see *The CFIDS Chronicle* or call the CFIDS Information Line. Also please refer to Appendix B.

Definition, causes, treatments and prognosis of CFIDS have been reprinted with permission from the *CFIDS Chronicle.*

Why a Name Such As CFIDS?

Chronic Fatigue and Immune Dysfunction Syndrome is an utterly confusing name that *I refuse to accept.* **Come on AMA!** *Can't you come up with a* ***BETTER name?*** **AIDS is not called Chronic Fatigue AIDS Dysfunction,** yet we suffer and are disabled like these poor souls, although CFIDS is not deadly. We will have to leave this statement open for debate. To me, a more specific name such as **Neuro-Immune Disorder** would be a more justifiable name for this disease.

Some of the feelings that CFIDS survivors experience are: we are dying, we are being ignored by most people, and we have lost everything, including the simple ability to work. This disease is like a slow death, because our brains are not functioning as they should.

Let us wake up to reality now! President Bill Clinton and our government and the medical profession need to *open their eyes and realize that* ***we have an epidemic on our hands—America's unknown epidemic.*** If we keep ignoring Chronic Fatigue and Immune Dysfunction the way the government ignored AIDS in the early 1980s, *we will have another monstrous disaster.* It does not make *sense* at all. We must fund more research *now.* Not only will early funding help us find a cure sooner, but it also will save money in the long run.

What will it take for the government to look at CFIDS seriously? Yes, AIDS is a devastating disease, but so is CFIDS. What makes things worse for CFIDS sufferers is that CFIDS *has not yet been acknowledged enough!* Families are not well informed, and most people, including medical professionals, do not understand CFIDS because of the lack of information available to the general public.

THERE IS NO EXCUSE FOR IGNORANCE!

The empty, lonely moments go on, with hope, that the **government will soon hear the cries of CFIDS sufferers.** Perhaps when the medical costs of CFIDS become an even larger burden on the government, CFIDS will not only be recognized, but also understood enough to be *acknowledged as a serious problem,* and *something will be done to bring this epidemic under control!*

Children and CFIDS

CFIDS also affects our children. If, as a parent or a responsible guardian, you are raising a child who is weak, ill, or cannot concentrate, has swollen glands, major mood swings, and/or sleep disturbances, your child may suffer from CFIDS. CFIDS is a multi-symptomatic disease. Please refer to the Chronic Fatigue Institute Questionnaire in Appendix B. It will help you recognize that your child may be suffering from CFIDS. Please, if your child is often ill, see a qualified, open-minded doctor who does not prescribe antibiotics freely. It is extremely important that your doctor diagnose the disease correctly and quickly start a proper treatment program.

Specialists on the treatment of children with CFIDS can be reached through The Chronic Fatigue and Immune Dysfunction Association of America

Personal Observations About the Cause of CFIDS

Antibiotics have certainly saved many lives, and thank God we have them, but we now know that overuse of antibiotics can cause other medical problems. One of the problems is Candida. I was given too many antibiotics—plain and simple, too many. Years back, we did not know that supplementing antibiotics with acidophillus would make it less harmful to us. Also, years ago, we did not know the devastating affect of mercury amalgam fillings in our teeth. Mercury weakens our immune system even further. With an already weakened immune system, and our terribly polluted environment (pesticides, food coloring, food preservatives, animal hormones, etc.), our bodies are open doors for viruses, colds, fungi, and infections. All of these things overload our immune system to the point of burnout.

Yes, my CFIDS started with mononucleosis, but I ask myself, why did I not recover? One answer to that question is that my body was already in a weakened state. Stress and malnutrition in my childhood, too many antibiotics, mercury fillings, and untreated Candida had all impacted my immune system. This enabled many viruses to invade my body. I had parasites that went untreated for years. Now, I have been diagnosed with Herpes I, CVM, Herpes VI, and the Epstein-Barr virus. These viruses act in a vicious cycle. They are dormant for some time, reactivating themselves with the presence of stress or illness. For example: I get Herpes I every 6 to 8 weeks; I feel like I have the flu, get blisters inside and outside of my mouth, a slight fever, swollen glands, and terrible head, body, and neck pain. These symptoms usually lessen within one week. The other viruses I was tested for also activate randomly, never giving the body a chance to recuperate fully. I would say from my own observations that CFIDS is a **Herpes strain virus infection!** Unless we strengthen our immune systems so they can fight back, we cannot get well.

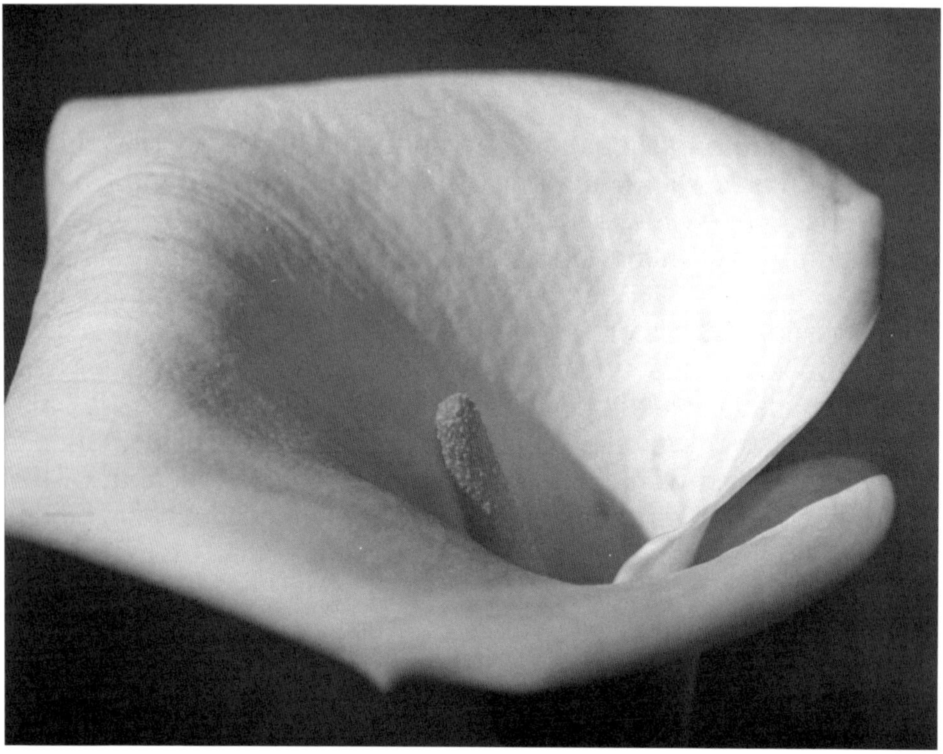

Photo by Thea.

Chapter Three

Symptoms of CFIDS

Suicide and CFIDS

The author of *CFIDS the Crippler,* Mike Culbert DN.,D.C., writes that eventually CFIDS will put more people in the hospital than AIDS and cancer combined. Many of us know very well what it is like to live with CFIDS. Yes, it is tough and, at times, almost unbearable. It always saddens me to hear, read, or find out that again a CFIDS sufferer has committed suicide. At times, I feel, "How can I go on living this way?" I have to. We all have our breaking points. It takes all we have in us to keep going with this horrible body disease. Equally as devastating is that this illness is not even properly acknowledged. Some still say to this day that it is a psychological disease! Unbelievable, but true.

How ignorant and sad, because it is America's unknown epidemic. It really is no surprise, as sad as it is for me to write, that some CFIDS survivors just give up. Many of us have lost almost everything. People do not understand us. Our pain is almost constant, and our emotional stability and life are in limbo. Our partners are not able to cope with us and neither, at times, are our families and friends. By the same token, we CFIDS survivors often have a hard time coping with our lives.

This does not excuse any one of us who kill ourselves. It just absolutely devastates me when I learn of the death of another CFIDS sufferer. We must endure. I personally plea to each one of you who reads this book: take this illness for what it is. Do not despair. Reach out for help before giving up your precious life. Keep remembering—there is **always** hope.

Restless Leg Syndrome

Restless Leg Syndrome is a neurological disorder caused by an imbalance in the brain. It is a common problem among CFIDS survivors. It takes hours to go to sleep, and you just keep moving your legs. Dr. Goldstein prescribes Klonopin for this condition, and it has helped me.

There are some things that you can do if you suffer from Restless Leg Syndrome. Try wearing silk pajamas, wiggling your legs before going to bed, or soaking your feet in warm water. Also, cold weather can make Restless Leg Syndrome worse, so try sleeping with an electric blanket and wearing cotton socks to bed. Electric blankets have received much negative attention, and rightfully so, because electricity does affect our bodies. However, I have found that the warmth of an electric blanket on the lowest setting helps me sleep better and the symptoms of Restless Leg Syndrome are relieved. Reducing stress and avoiding large meals before bedtime may also give you some relief. You should also check to make sure that you do not have anemia, as this condition can also cause Restless Leg Syndrome.

Parasites

Do most of us have parasites, even in the United States? The answer is a surprising YES! Unless we get rid of these parasites, we cannot get well. A simple stool test can detect parasites, but sometimes they are overlooked. Some of the symptoms of parasite invasion include feeling tired all of the time and constant nausea.

People can pick up these unwelcome invaders from restaurant food that has been contaminated by infected workers. Improperly cooked food can also lead to transmission of parasites, including tapeworm from fish. Roundworms and salmonella are other common sickness-causing organisms.

Many times, illnesses that have gone undiagnosed for years, and are seemingly unrelated to the intestinal tract, disappear after natural treatment for parasite infection. Even mild infestations may cause bothersome health problems. Case in point: some doctors found that many patients with Candida Albicans cannot get rid of the Candida until their bodies are rid of the parasites. Indeed, many people unwittingly host parasite parties within their own bodies!

Fortunately, nature provides many substances that are the sworn enemies of parasites. Health-conscious consumers can turn to herbal cleansers designed to nutritionally support the body in its efforts to evict these uninvited guests. Such cleansers are perfect marriages of time-honored Chinese tradition and Western knowledge.

Insomnia

Where should I start with this agonizing symptom called insomnia, which is so common among CFIDS survivors? Insomnia is terrible to have. Most people go to sleep after going to bed and wake up feeling refreshed. This is certainly not the case when one has CFIDS. Not only do we feel exhausted during the day, but when we want to go sleep at night, we cannot, either due to Restless Leg Syndrome, general body pain, or the fact that our minds keep racing. This is very annoying. And even on the odd night that we get a good night's sleep, we do not wake up feeling refreshed. If I did not take Klonapin, I probably would not sleep at all, or almost not at all for days at a time.

Temporomandibular Joint Syndrome and Related Myofacial Pain

Temporomandibular Joint Syndrome (TMJ) is very common among CFIDS survivors. Luckily, with newly developed high-tech instrumentation, the ability to successfully diagnose and treat TMJ and related problems without surgery has made a major jump forward. However, with some extremely severe cases where bony defects result from advanced osteoarthritic destruction of the jaw, surgery is still the only option. It is also possible that symptoms may be caused by some undiagnosed medical or dental problem, other than the temporomandibular joint. For instance, once my teeth and partial dentures where in correct alignment, my TMJ got a lot better. Also, I've found that osteopathic treatments helped greatly.

Many patients have already been from one specialist to another, trying to find the underlying cause for their apparently bizarre symptoms. Some are referred by physicians, others by dentists, psychiatrists, and other health-related specialists, to explore the possibility of TMJ or related muscle dysfunction as a possible cause of their problems.

Generally, it is found that patients suffering from TMJ and related muscular problems experience some or all of the following symptoms.

Candida—Fungus Infection

Candida is a very common symptom associated with CFIDS. It is usually brought on by an overuse of antibiotics. Antibiotics kill both good and bad bacteria in our digestive systems. Candida can affect either the entire body or specific parts, and it is very difficult to bring under control. To replace the good flow of flora, it is advised to take acidophillus.

If you suffer from a fungus infection in the vagina, over-the-counter products are now available. For severe cases, always consult your doctor. He may put you on anti-fungal medication and a strict diet. Henry Hoegerman, M.D., kindly contributed an article on Candida. You can find it in Appendix A.

Hypothyroidism

Almost everybody with CFIDS has hypothyroidism. It takes a T3, T4, T7, and TSH profile to determine how your thyroid is performing. I have to take syntroid for my thyroid. Many symptoms are connected with a low thyroid, such as low energy, low resistance to colds and flu, low body temperature, insomnia, low appetite, and headaches. It is very important to have your thyroid checked. The test is expensive, but worth every penny. You cannot get well if your thyroid is functioning low. Likewise, a high functioning thyroid (hyperthyroidism) can also cause many of problems.

Brain Fog

My brain. My brain. What is going on? As so often in the past, I feel as if my brain is dying. It is as though my head has been disconnected from my body. I hardly ever feel a clear mind. My head hurts, my brain feels inflamed; so does my entire skull. Sometimes, it feels as if lightning is going through the right side of my brain. My muscles are twitching all over my body. I am actually afraid that someone might call. Any type of noise hurts. My windows are closed, my blinds are shut. This has been going on for years. When will it stop? God, please give me my brain back—**please!**

I write, instinctively, a few lines at a time. Sometimes, I feel panic-stricken, not knowing what is happening with my brain. I feel nauseated and totally exhausted. I cannot even get dressed, not today.

There are too many days like that, and my bed is the only way out. I will turn my telephone off. Too ill to talk to anybody. I just keep quiet. What else can I do?

I keep hoping that tomorrow I will have more energy.

Whatever I say or hear, I forget it almost instantly. That is why I keep a tape recorder beside my phone. This way, I can tape conversations and when I feel better, I listen to the tapes. It also cuts down on my loneliness when I play the tape later. I replay the recording—especially if it is from a loved one. It keeps me company this way. This is the only way that I can have company most of the time.

When I am feeling this bad, I have to cut out all family problems, as my entire body feels inflamed and my nervous system is frazzled. I cannot watch TV, listen to the radio, or read right now. I just have to lie down in bed, waiting, waiting, and waiting until my brain is functioning better. No wonder some of us end up in mental institutions if we are not diagnosed correctly. Right now, everything bothers me. I made myself a cup of coffee. It helps me write a few more lines.

The headaches are a challenge, too. When we lose control of the brain, we lose control of our bodies, as well. My legs keep moving, my body wants to rest, so does my mind, but how?

I wonder why my brain feels like this? Could it be that these are toxins from the viruses, Candida, and bacteria in my body? Is a chronic inflammation or swelling of the brain secondary to the overload of toxins in my body? I wonder if this will ever stop, if I'll ever be able to think straight again or to fully remember conversations. At times, I have been told that I repeat myself. I feel embarrassed by this. More so before I knew that I had CFIDS. Now, I try very hard to just accept these comments.

Who am I? Thea is my name, but Thea is not Thea anymore. For now, all I can do is wait for a better day. Pray, pray, pray, and pray. At least I do have a room and my bed. Many precious souls do not even have that. Their only home is the street. No blankets to keep them warm, hardly enough food to survive, and a constant feeling of rejection. So I should not complain. I know this, but it is hard not to complain. At times, I break down and cry.

Allergies

Allergies are symptoms of immune depletion. Find out what you are allergic to and do something about it. CFIDS is toxic enough. You do not need any other burdens on the immune system. When I was tested for allergies, I was not surprised to find that I was allergic to sixty-four of the seventy-two environmental substances for which I was tested. This was in 1976. Later, in 1989, when I was at the clinic in Mexico, I was tested for food allergies. Again, a high count of allergies to food, spices, food colorings, and medicines. It is a must to avoid anything that you are allergic to, if you can.

Mercury Fillings

In 1992, Henry Hoegerman, M.D., suggested that I have the fillings in my teeth changed to a different material. Needless to say, any mercury fillings are very toxic. However, I was surprised to find that the material used in white fillings can cause problems, too. My dentist, who specializes in the removal of mercury fillings, also advised me to have all the mercury fillings from my teeth removed and some teeth pulled.

My dentist tested me for toxic levels from the mercury, and the levels were extremely high. He had to do the procedure slowly. There is a certain technique involved that costs a great deal of money. The worst part was that my upper eyeteeth had had root canals, and he could not save the other upper teeth. He suggested dentures, since partials would not have had any support without eyeteeth. It took me six months to decide what to do. I finally agreed to have dentures. My beautiful teeth had to go, and I had to wear dentures. I cannot seem to adjust to them, and they make me feel older than I really am. Of course, although I hate wearing them, I must admit that I am glad that there are dentures. What would I do if they did not exist? My thinking at the time was that I had to make a choice—look good or get healthier—and I made the choice to get healthier.

Now, three years later, I regret very much letting the dentist pull all of my upper teeth. It turns out that the eyeteeth could have been replaced with dental implants, and they could have held a partial denture in place. To pull my teeth was a drastic mistake. Please, if you have a problem with your teeth, get a second and third opinion. I wish I had!

Fibromyalgia

Many researchers believe that CFIDS and Fibromyalgia are the same disease. They certainly share symptoms, and both excel in broadcasting pain throughout the body. For me, the mornings have always been the worst. Neck, shoulders, and head all throb so hard that it feels as if they may just fall apart from the pain. One way to be sure if you are afflicted with Fibromyalgia is to look for certain "trigger points."

There are support groups for people who suffer with Fibromyalgia and a lot that you can do about this painful condition. Hot and cold packs, mineral ice, light exercise, and various vitamins all help to relieve the pain.

It is common knowledge that Fibromyalgia is one of the most painful forms of arthritis pain there is. Spasms and nodules of pain appear between the shoulder blades and other parts of the body. Accupressure is a fairly effective aid for many, while others take anti-inflammatory medicine, as well as antidepressants. I have also tried the TENS unit which, if you don't know, is a small computer-generated neurotransmitter that sends a low electronic current into the nerves that are sending pain signals to the brain. In many cases, the TENS procedure can interrupt the pain transmission and provide some symptomatic relief.

Changes in the weather can be particularly difficult for those with Fibromyalgia. In my case, I find that dry, warm weather seems to be ideal. Those afflicted with CFIDS and Fibromyalgia are also nearly always deprived of sleep. For many, antidepressants seem to help. Dr. Goldstein gave me an I.V. for fibromyalgia which really helped.

Metal Toxicity

When lead is deposited in the bones, these deposits take exactly the same pattern as calcium deposits. If both lead and calcium are present, the bone is more likely to take up the lead, because the lead compounds are less soluble than calcium phosphates. But if extra calcium is given before lead, less lead is taken up by the bones and more is found in the stomach on its way to being excreted. This finding suggests a high calcium diet to prevent excessive lead absorption. One also wonders whether lead deposits in the bones are sometimes mistaken for calcium deposits in x-rays.

A Japanese researcher, Giro Obara, experimented with several treatments for tetra-ethyl lead poisoning. He points out that acute tetra-ethyl lead poisoning brings on more mental effects than does inorganic lead, perhaps because it vaporizes and is then rapidly absorbed into the organism. Vitamin B1 and sodium thiosulfate each helped alleviate the poisoning symptoms, he found, but large doses of vitamin C had the greatest effect by far as an antidote.

Obara also measured the lactic acid and sugar content of the blood, and found that, shortly after poisoning, these values rose sharply only to decrease quickly, resulting in hypoglycemia. Apparently, when the poison reaches the liver, it releases glycogen, causing the initial rise, but the continuing action of the lead results in the eventual lowering of glycogen by the liver. Measurements showed liver and muscle glycogen to be almost entirely absent at the end of the experiment.

Further tests showed that the poisoning reduces the liver's ability to form new glycogen from added glucose, but that vitamin B1, vitamin C, and sodium thiosulfate all helped to neutralize that effect.

Lead poisoning is only one example of what metal toxicity can do to you. It is of utmost importance to have the metal balance in your body checked. Usually, a urine analysis and hair analysis provide the proper information to determine if you have too much metal in your body. Ask your health-care provider about these easy, yet necessary tests.

Low Blood Pressure

Late in 1995, The Journal of the American Medical Association reported strong links between CFIDS and a common abnormality in the way the body regulates blood pressure. Many patients respond well with increased fluid and salt intake and, sometimes, a drug to regulate blood pressure. Researchers at Johns Hopkins Hospital in Baltimore carried out the study.

"The finding of a link between the two conditions is very solid," Dr. Hugh Calkins, the senior author of this study, said in an interview. But he also cautioned that treatment findings were preliminary and needed to be verified in a larger study conducted under more scientifically rigid criteria before it is widely applied among the millions who have CFIDS.

Hypotension commonly occurs when the central nervous system's autonomic portion, which controls heart rate and blood pressure response, misinterprets the body's need during periods of upright posture and sends a message to the heart to slow down and lower blood pressure. Such a response is the opposite of what the body needs at such times, according to the researchers.

We have to keep in mind that this particular kind of low blood pressure cannot be detected by standard blood pressure tests. It is instead discerned by tilting the patient at a certain degree angle to the floor to stimulate standing for a long period of time, which commonly brings on the low blood pressure response.

I Am

Unconditionally

Loving

and

Accepting

of Myself

Every Day

and

In Every

Way!

Chapter Four

Coping Skills: Living with CFIDS

Acceptance

One of the hardest things to accept is having an illness for which, as of this writing, there is no known 100%-sure cure. I may be wrong, but to my knowledge, once someone has CFIDS for more than five years, the likelihood of relapse is very high.

When I was first diagnosed in 1989, I was happy to know that this long, unknown illness *had a name.* But then reality hit me, and I realized that the illness I have is extremely difficult to treat. It takes a lot of discipline to learn to accept the fact that you have an illness in which your body controls you and not the other way around. Does it make sense to feel sorry for ourselves and let life go by, or is it not wiser to accept the fact as it is and live life the best way we can.

There are millions of people in this world who have an illness. Regardless of the diagnosis, it is not easy for anyone to be ill. Needless to say, having CFIDS is difficult to take perhaps, since not much is known about this illness; and there are many people who don't even know about CFIDS, including many members of the medical community. Not only do we suffer from this illness, but we are not even accepted by society yet. This makes accepting that you have CFIDS unbearable at times. I find that praying is the most powerful way to heal the soul, to calm the heart, and to help me get through the day. Once we accept the truth as it is, we stop fighting life in an unfulfilled way. We cannot stop a big powerful ocean wave from reaching the shores, so is it not wisest to rise with the current? I believe it is.

Forgiveness

Unless we learn to forgive, we can never find peace with ourselves. It would be easy for me to hate or blame everybody who treated me badly or the war, which made life so difficult to bear. It would be easy to hate the doctors who for years misdiagnosed me. Perhaps some people deserve to be hated by me. Then I ask myself—who would this benefit? The answer is NOBODY! Christ forgave those who turned against him and even *prayed* for them.

In all my years in this great universe, I have tried to forgive everybody. If I do not forgive someone, that unhealthy feeling and negative energy can turn into hate, and hate would only prevent me from getting better. I learned a long time ago that praying for those who hurt me is the best thing for both of us. **I do not want that bad energy in my body.** Forgiveness is healthy. Let us remember that. There is too much hate in this world. I would rather forgive and love someone. We all have a choice in dealing with people who hurt us. Try to make the right choice for you.

My Precious, Supporting Family

I haven't really talked much about my children and grandchildren. It is almost too painful to get into this subject. I lost so much time with my children, and we have gone through so much despair. This is why this subject is the most difficult to put into words. I will try to keep it short.

CFIDS survivors know how it feels. Not only do patients of CFIDS feel helpless, but so does everyone around them. I want desperately to be able to care for my family; to be a good mother and wife, as well as a good friend and sister. I pushed myself every day to the limit. I did not want to give in to the energy depletion and body pain, not to mention all of the other CFIDS symptoms. This was a big mistake, because the body can take only so much.

My family was always very supportive, and I'm sure they knew how quickly I tired, probably more than I'm aware of. My love for them was there emotionally, but, physically, there was no way I could show them how much I loved them. During my illness, everyone pitched in. I can remember Ingrid and Elly baking, washing, and cleaning, hardly ever complaining. They both respected the effects of this unknown illness on me since it started, in 1970.

All the while, I kept wondering to myself, *"What is happening?"* My fantasy life was now only a faint memory. I was afraid that I was dying, but too afraid to tell anyone.

In 1986 I was unable to be with my daughter during the birth of my grandson Ryan. Ingrid gave birth to Ryan on the second floor of the hospital while I was on the third floor, receiving electric shock treatments again. Ingrid must have felt so abandoned by me. This is sad. I have no memory of Ryan's birth at all. On the sixth shock treatment I went into cardiac arrest. Happily, I was able to be with my other grandsons' births and videotaped and photographed these joyous events. I felt so filled with emotion that tears of joy streamed down my face. It always took days to recover from any activity, but I really did not care. As long as I could participate in my family's lives I was happy.

When I was finally diagnosed with CFIDS, my family and friends kept asking me what it was. The questions are now being answered, and it is helping that all of the people who are closest to me finally understand what I've been going through all these years.

While many were especially supportive, others had a very hard time seeing me so helpless and that, in turn, made them feel helpless. When we are feeling our lowest, it is then that we must pick ourselves up and make the best of what is given to us by our Creator.

Truly Understanding

When a loved one becomes ill, we feel helpless. That helpless feeling turns into anger, frustration, and, eventually, an overwhelming feeling that the situation has become impossible.

I know. I've been, and still go, through it. Some can cope better than others. Ingrid was able to cope with the help of her husband, yet Elly could not. For six years, I thought that Elly and Mike didn't love me anymore. Then, I realized that they truly did, but they were so sick and tired of seeing me sick that their only survival was to almost cut me out of their lives. Deep down in my heart, I knew they cared. Mike helped me in the camera store. He operated the photo lab by himself, and Santa Barbara Camera & Thea's Photo Express quickly became known as one of the finest photo-finishers around, thanks to Mike's hard work.

Now, we are very close again. It feels so good. I know that it was just as hard for Elly and Mike to cope as it was for me.

It is truly difficult enough to be sick, but to not be acknowledged or respected anymore is even more painful. Wouldn't it be great to always be supportive of each other?

Let me tell you what having CFIDS is.

You feel like you have the flu all of the time, for years. People think that you are lazy. You can't sleep, and you are exhausted. Every bone in your body aches, and you feel so confused and hopeless that, at times, it scares you. Your family cannot understand why you cannot make it to their parties as you lie in bed, totally exhausted.

You are so tired. Depression sets in. Your glands are swollen and you feel dizzy, nauseated, and as if you are in a constant fog. Your vision changes, you have panic attacks, anxiety, memory loss, and you can't even manage to balance your checkbook. Every day, there is an inner hope that this monstrous illness will go away, but instead you wake up feeling the same as you did yesterday.

You tell people that you are tired. They respond by saying that they are tired, too, that everyone gets tired, but they manage to take care of their responsibilities regardless. What can you say? They do not understand that CFIDS is an illness. It is an actual immune dysfunction. If you felt like this, wouldn't you appreciate a loving, caring hand? A supportive heart? Someone who cares and understands and believes you?

Please, if you know someone who is ill, give them your love and support. Love can work wonders. Understanding provides dignity. Support lifts self-esteem. It is hard enough to deal with the illness without being judged and misunderstood or, even, ignored.

Wouldn't it be wonderful if we could just say "I love you" to one person each day? With that in mind, I would like to end this chapter by saying, "I LOVE YOU."

Relationships and CFIDS

We all long for someone in our lives who can give us love and companionship, whether it be a mate or a special friend. This person can help us overcome the obstacles in life and make that which can seem so overwhelming more bearable.

CFIDS changes all that, because of its crippling effect on the entire body and mind. It is hard, *very hard*, to admit to yourself that it is NOT easy being around you. One moment you feel happy and the next, exhausted. Ups and downs are a constant way of life. How can a loved one keep up with this? If the situation were reversed, I think that I would be able to, because love is stronger than anything in life. But so many of us cannot cope with someone else's illness. It is no wonder that so many relationships where one partner has CFIDS cannot seem to survive. I ask myself, "Are those who cannot support us emotionally with this illness selfish?" I do not think so. Sometimes, it may be that they love you so very much, they cannot cope with seeing you hurting. It is very sad that there is not enough understanding to teach us how to cope with sick partners. Life is so short, and love is so precious. Love is the greatest gift we can receive and give, yet it is thrown away because we cannot cope with ill people. Why not go to counseling? Is it not better to spend just one or two hours a day with the person you love, learning to cope, than to not love at all? Life can be very lonely, but I try to fill the loneliness with positive experiences.

Setting Goals

Knowing very well how it feels to live with CFIDS, I am desperately trying to make the best of this situation. Setting goals provides a feeling of accomplishment. For example, I signed up with The American College of Nutritional Medicine to get my Ph.D. in Philosophy and Nutrition. I have no idea when I'll finish my Ph.D., but doing homework once in a while and sending it off to be graded makes me feel better. I got my first test back, and I failed it! But I actually did much better than I had hoped to do. I will take the test again. That becomes another goal. I am a person who needs to set goals, otherwise I start to think about CFIDS and feel sorry for myself. This does not do anyone any good. It is important for me to not be disappointed if I fail at something. Rather, I know that I tried in spite of having CFIDS, and I am proud of myself. It is easy to fall into the trap of feeling sorry for myself; therefore, it is important to look at CFIDS as a challenge.

For instance, when I was in the mental institution in 1972, I developed a new game, which I named "Challenge your IQ." I got it copyrighted in 1977. This was a large feat for me to accomplish, especially considering that I was in the mental institution at the time. Developing this game gave me a very valuable sense of self-worth and accomplishment. I do not think that everyone needs to go out and invent and copyright something. Doing something, anything, that will increase your sense of accomplishment will also lift your spirits and help you cope.

I do believe that it is our attitude in life that either makes us succeed or feel trapped and hopeless. That is why goal-setting is so important. Keeping a diary has helped me a lot, too. This is an easy way to take inventory of my life. The diary shows me whether I am on the right track, or if I might want to change my direction.

The bottom line is, yes, we are ill, but let us enjoy the things we can do and forget those that, at this time, we cannot do. I try to use CFIDS to learn about humanity and have compassion for others.

Whatever happened with my game, "Challenge Your IQ"? Frankly, nothing. This is too bad, because it really is a fascinating game. It could even be a television game show. One thing at a time. Perhaps the game will come to reality one day. This would make me very happy.

Be Kind to Yourself

I am a type A personality, and I have a terrible time with CFIDS, but I am learning to listen to the signal to stop. If I do not, I pay a high price.

Stop—relax—be kind to yourself. Most of what I am writing is from personal experience, and I am trying to alert you to some of the problems that may happen to you, so that you can make better decisions on how or what you need to do to make your life with this disease as easy as possible. It is not my intention to preach to anyone. I just want to spare anyone from some of the agony that I have gone through.

I have joined a CFIDS activist group and am currently writing and doing television shows in order to spread the word. If you wish to be a part of this group, and we do need help, please contact the CFIDS Society. We need all the help we can possibly get. You can find the address and phone number in Appendix B.

Positive Imaging

Positive imaging can do wonders. I realize how difficult it is to keep positive images in our minds, but it is something that we must do in order to recover. For instance, when I was hospitalized in 1990 with encephalitis, I was near death. I covered my hospital room doors and walls with photographs that I had taken. This way, instead of feeling the constant agony of pain, I was able to think of where I was when I took those pictures. I thought about the aperture and film speed that I used and the time-consuming challenge of composing a photograph to my liking. I remembered how wonderful it had been to receive six international gold medals and the many other awards I received for my photographs. I remembered how honored I felt when I saw my photos in magazines. This positive imaging was a way to give me hope. I kept thinking that, one day, I would be able to do it all again. Before I go to bed, I imagine myself going dancing or to the symphony, or maybe to a ballet, an opera, or a play. Sometimes, I imagine myself playing tennis again. I never give up. I try my hardest to always participate in activities with my wonderful family, going to birthday parties and other events when I can.

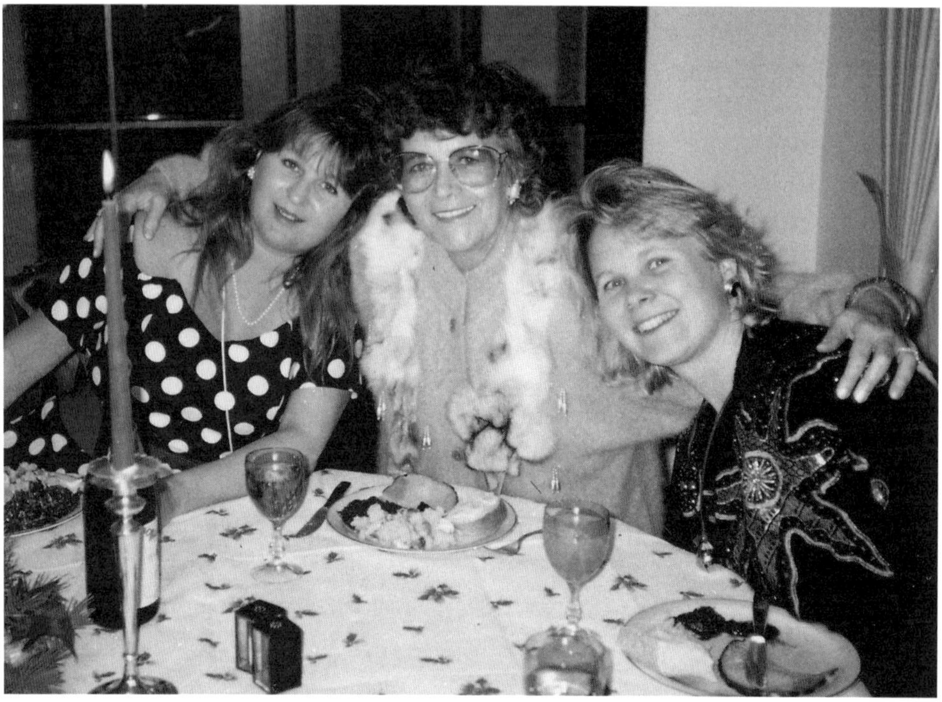

My dear daughters Elly and Ingrid with me, Christmas 1993.

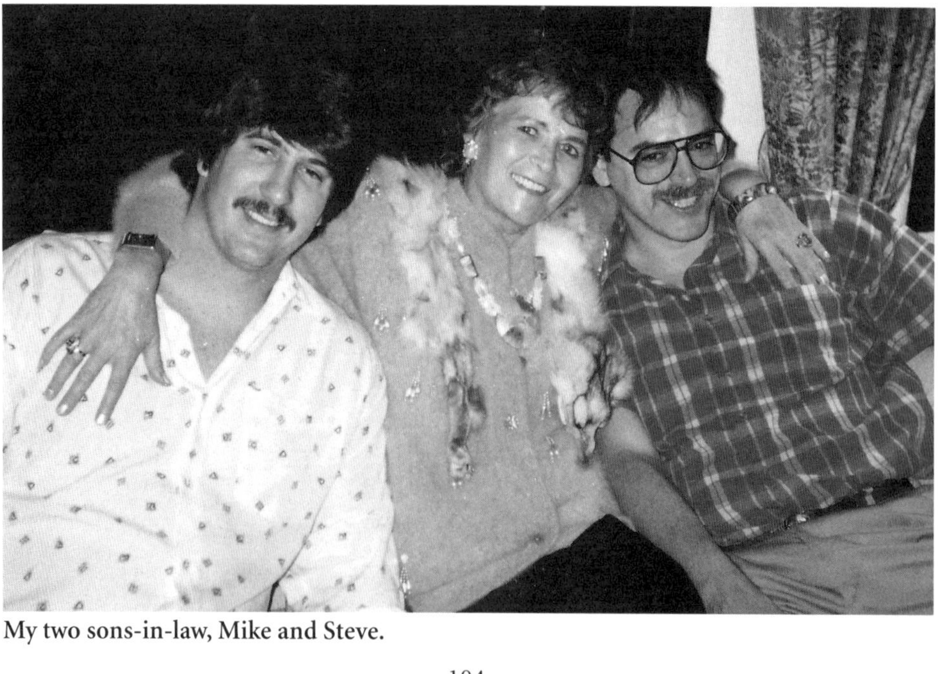

My two sons-in-law, Mike and Steve.

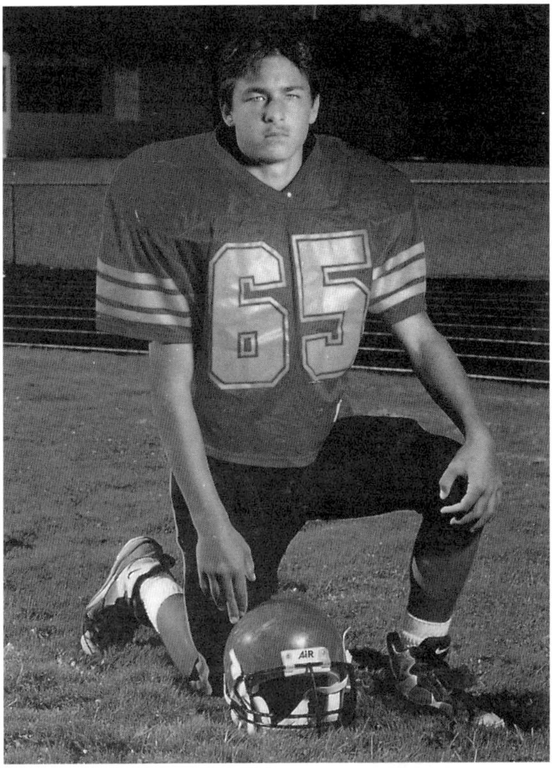

My grandchildren Shane (above) and Chris (right) Prukop, Elly and Mike's children.

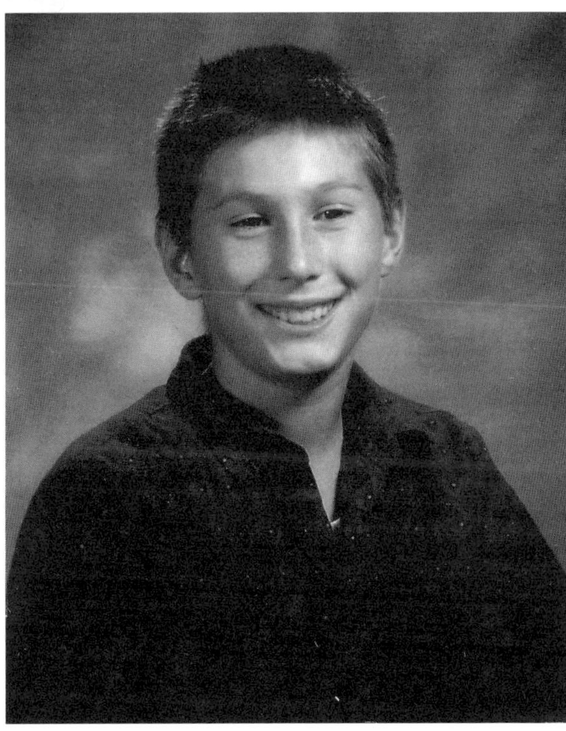

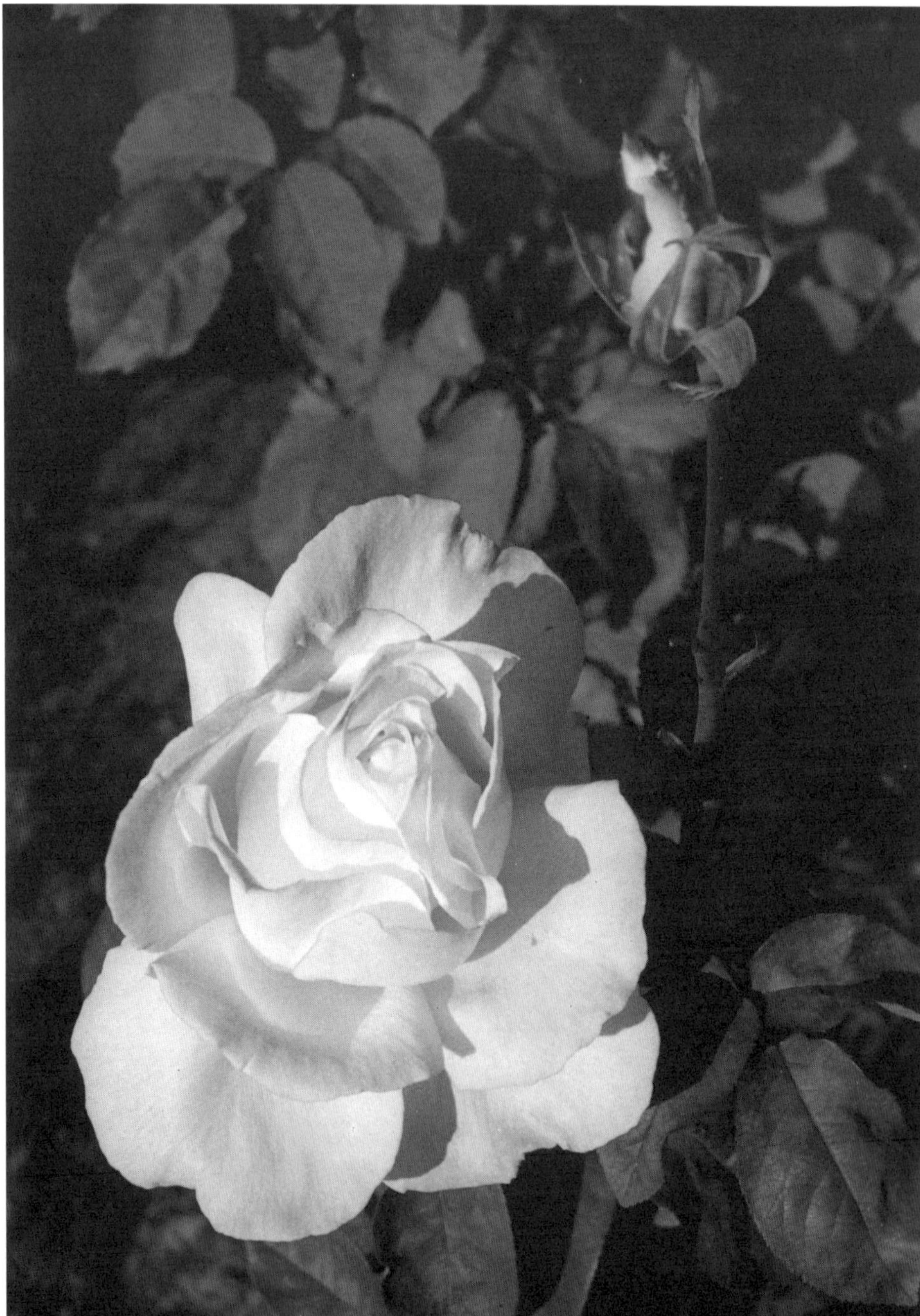

Photo by Thea.

Chapter Five

Self-Treatments

Coffee Enemas and Colonics

I feel that both of these are indispensable. Coffee, when you drink it, is very toxic, but taken rectally, it helps to stimulate the liver and get rid of toxins in the body faster. I have a coffee enema about once a week. I do my own colonic with the colonic board. Most of the time, I liquefy three heads of garlic in a pint of water and add it to my colonic water bucket. I also add about one teaspoon of cayenne pepper. The pepper brings on a more effective bowel movement. Garlic is a powerful detoxifier. It takes about forty-five minutes, but it is well worth the effort. When I give myself a colonic, I skip the coffee enema. I also find that taking coffee enemas helps lessen my headaches. Please refer to the article on the colon in this section for more information.

Yoga

Yoga is a very relaxing form of exercise for muscle toning and energy. It is not difficult to learn and, as an added bonus for CFIDS patients, is not strenuous. I purchased a yoga videotape set from the CFIDS Buyer's Club. So, whenever I feel like it, I do yoga, enjoying it.

Deep Breathing

Breathing costs nothing, yet it is very important. It feeds oxygen to our entire system, prevents damage to our cells, and gives us energy. Try to breathe in and out deeply for ten breaths about three times a day. It is also very relaxing.

Since CFIDS patients are frequently very inactive due to the constant need for rest, our lungs do not get the benefit of deep breathing that is so very important. I try to deep breathe wherever I can, be it in the car, in bed, or in the shower. It is easy to do and so important for our recovery that there is no excuse for not doing it!

Exercise

Exercise can be difficult for CFIDS sufferers as, in many cases, we can barely muster up enough energy to get through the day, let alone manage to work in an exercise routine. Some type of movement, even lifting your arms a few times a day, can be beneficial, as the body needs movement to help increase blood flow to the brain and all through the body. Exercise is important, very important, but please do it carefully. If you feel just a little tired, stop! Try again in a day or two. We all hear that we should exercise and that it is very beneficial for everyone. This is not always the case with CFIDS patients. Exercise can actually make us feel worse if we overdo it. At times, two minutes of walking is enough. Only you can know when to stop. I walk or stretch when I feel up to it, but I've noticed that if I don't use common sense, it is counter-productive. I am easy on myself. I walk, but not for long. Ten minutes is usually a good amount of time.

At the very least, if you cannot exercise, try using a shower-head massage. This also seems to provide benefits in improved circulation.

Fasting

There are many types of fasts. One type that I do not believe in is the water-only fast. I may be wrong, but for me, that is too much for the body to go through. Fasting, if done correctly, is very healing.

When fasting, try to get extra rest. It is of utmost importance that you get advice from your health-care provider, including the length of time that you should fast and what kind of fast you should follow. I usually fast from one to three days and include a detoxification supplement to help my body get rid of toxins. Positive thinking while you fast is also beneficial.

Sunshine

Sunshine gives us Vitamins C and D and re-energizes us; thus, it is important for our overall well-being. Of course, too much sunshine is harmful. Although a tan looks nice, it is a result of damage done to the skin. CFIDS patients should try to avoid too much sun. But don't avoid it altogether.

At times, when I feel low in spirit and feel that everybody can take a vacation except for me, I put on my bikini, put sun block lotion on, lie down on my lawn chair, and pretend that I am on vacation. I try to look for a bird, or observe something in nature, and remind myself of the beauty that surrounds us all. Sometimes, having CFIDS, we forget about this free gift from God.

Stress

Stress is the one thing that CFIDS patients cannot afford. We need a calm life, as stable as possible. Try to be around people who understand what you are going through. And, by all means, join a support group if one is available. I use classical music to calm me down. I've also found that meditation and relaxation tapes help to relax me. I try to avoid anything stressful, but even things that are not stressful at all to others tend to be major steps for me and take a lot of effort. If I cannot do something, I have the tendency to get upset, which, in turn, becomes stress. I have found that the best way to handle stress is to not expect too much of myself, something that's easier said than done.

When I feel like I need a break, I try taking a warm bath or shower or giving myself a facial. Sometimes, I sit in the sun for a short time. I also find reading poems and praying very relaxing. Once in a while, I'll even have a foot bath or a massage. These things both relax and refresh me. My camera still provides me with a sense of purpose. Creating a good photograph is very rewarding. Try what you feel works best for you. We are all unique.

Redesigning Your Future

A famed minister once said, "Thoughts are things." Try to think of something that you can do to appreciate yourself. Could you brush your teeth? Go to the mailbox? If the answer is yes, then great! Do it, and then pat yourself on the back. Try not to think about what you cannot do; rather, concentrate on what you are able to do. Even if you can only lie in bed, don't be upset. Remember, you are a creation of God. You are special. There is no other person like you in the universe, and that is a miracle and a gift in itself.

Forgive yourself, love yourself and others unconditionally. You may feel that thinking positively or loving yourself is too difficult or not beneficial. I have been there and sometimes still am. One of the reasons why I am getting better is because I have disciplined myself to be more positive against all odds. I learned to love myself, as well as everyone around me. Believe me, I know. Remember, we are all survivors. We are all capable of redesigning our futures. As a matter of fact, CFIDS almost forces us to. It may not be easy, but it is definitely well worth the try.

Love

We must never choke the flow of love. To love is to give, and we are lucky to receive it. Love is special. We must do our best to not judge others, especially those in need and trouble. I believe that nobody is born bad. Reach out and give a helping hand. A smile or a nice remark can go such a long way.

Ingrid gave me a gift one day. It is a heart-shaped crystal, engraved "Your greatest gift to me is your love." This gift means so much to me; it has so much meaning.

Let's love each other as much as we are able. Hate only hurts us more. Love opens the doors to almost every possible situation. Love is healing. The vibration of love can heal almost anything. Love starts with loving ourselves first. Only then can we love others. Judging others and ourselves too harshly only shuts our spirit down. Then we close down. Try to keep the love flowing. Love is the greatest healer.

The Colon

It is frequently found that the refuse in the colon is from one to even ten days late in passing out, which means that the poisons that should have been eliminated are reabsorbed and thrown back into the bloodstream, then carried in the circulation to all parts of the body, thus poisoning it.

The colon is a sewage system, but by neglect and abuse, it becomes a cesspool. Taking our system for granted, thinking that it will take care of itself while we ignore it, is a mistake! When it is clean, we are well and happy. Let it stagnate, and it will distill the poisons of decay, fermentation, and putrefaction into the blood, poisoning the brain and nervous system so that we become mentally depressed and irritable.

It will poison the heart so that we are weak and listless. It poisons the lungs so that the breath is foul. It poisons the digestive organs so that we are distressed and bloated, and poisons the blood so that the skin is sallow and unhealthy. In short, every organ of the body is poisoned, and we age prematurely, look and feel old, and our joints become stiff and painful. The eyes are dull and the brain sluggish. The pleasure of life is gone.

Many grave diseases owe their existence to putrefaction of the colon. The fact that the symptoms of poisoning resulting from constipation do not appear at once is no evidence that injury is not done. It is no longer possible to ignore the importance of alimentary toxemia, or auto-intoxication, as a fact in the production of disease.

It may be said that almost every chronic disease known is directly or indirectly due to the influence of bacterial poisons absorbed from the intestines. The colon may be justly looked upon as a veritable Pandora's box, out of which comes more human misery and suffering—mental, moral, and physical—than from any other known source. Since we have CFIDS, it only makes sense that we rid ourselves of toxins through enemas and colonics. Needless to say, it is always best to consult your doctor before attempting an enema or a colonic.

Self-Hypnosis and Reassurance

Self-hypnosis works! Here's how to do it. Before going to bed at night, imagine the positive things you want to do tomorrow, even if it is something simple like taking a shower. Also, try to say a prayer. Then imagine something a little bigger. It will eventually happen.

Give yourself time to heal. It is hard, I know, and at times it may even feel impossible, but you must know that nothing is impossible.

It is easy to just give in because this crazy, confusing illness makes life so difficult. We are survivors, and great ones at that.

Going to bed feeling and thinking negative thoughts is very, very destructive to your recovery. It takes a lot of discipline to say, "I will feel good when I wake up tomorrow," knowing very well that this might not be the case. Regardless, you are still better off making and wishing for what you want. Over and over again. The subconscious mind is so powerful. Try to give it positive affirmation. You may be pleasantly surprised.

Grief

One of the most overlooked emotions for CFIDS sufferers is unresolved grief. CFIDS causes grief in itself. So a good cry relieves our despair and enables the body to take on a different energy flow. Allow yourself to grieve. Hit the pillow, scream, or take a walk, if you can. Otherwise, this grief will turn into anger and, eventually, depression.

Unemployment

CFIDS patients are eligible for state and government support. Check with your local Social Security Office and fill out the appropriate papers. Benefits could take up to a month to begin. If the Social Security Office denies your benefits, you may have to seek the services of an attorney. Remember, CFIDS has been recognized as a disease since 1988, and you are entitled to benefits.

My advice to you is to see an attorney right away—you will save a lot of time. The Social Security staff is usually very helpful and will assist you the best they can, but, at times, professional help not only saves you time, but since CFIDS is so exhausting, an attorney can do all the legwork for you. Just don't forget to ask for a quoted fee ahead of time and ask if they are familiar with CFIDS.

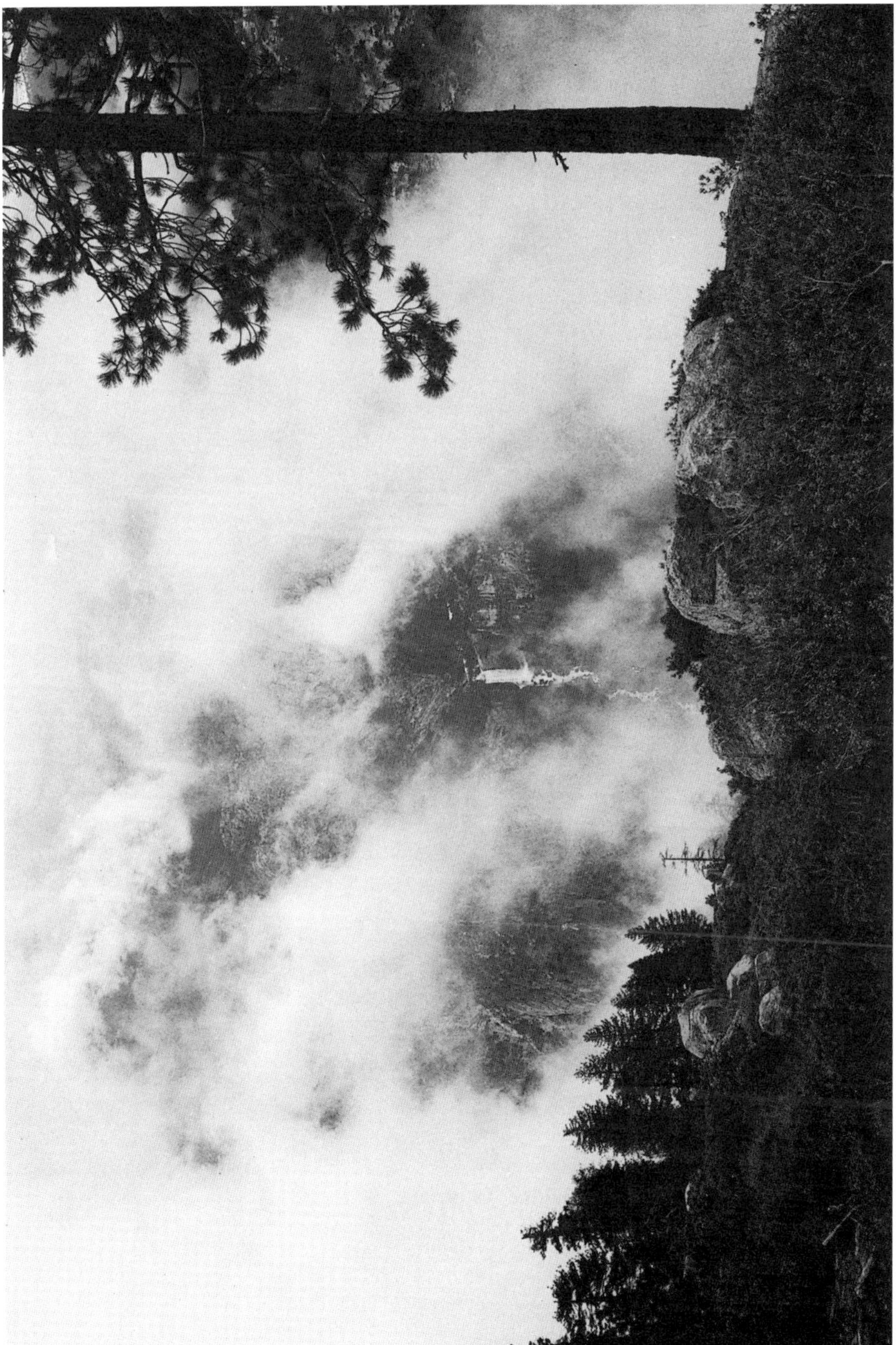

Photo by Thea. Zion Canyon, 1983.

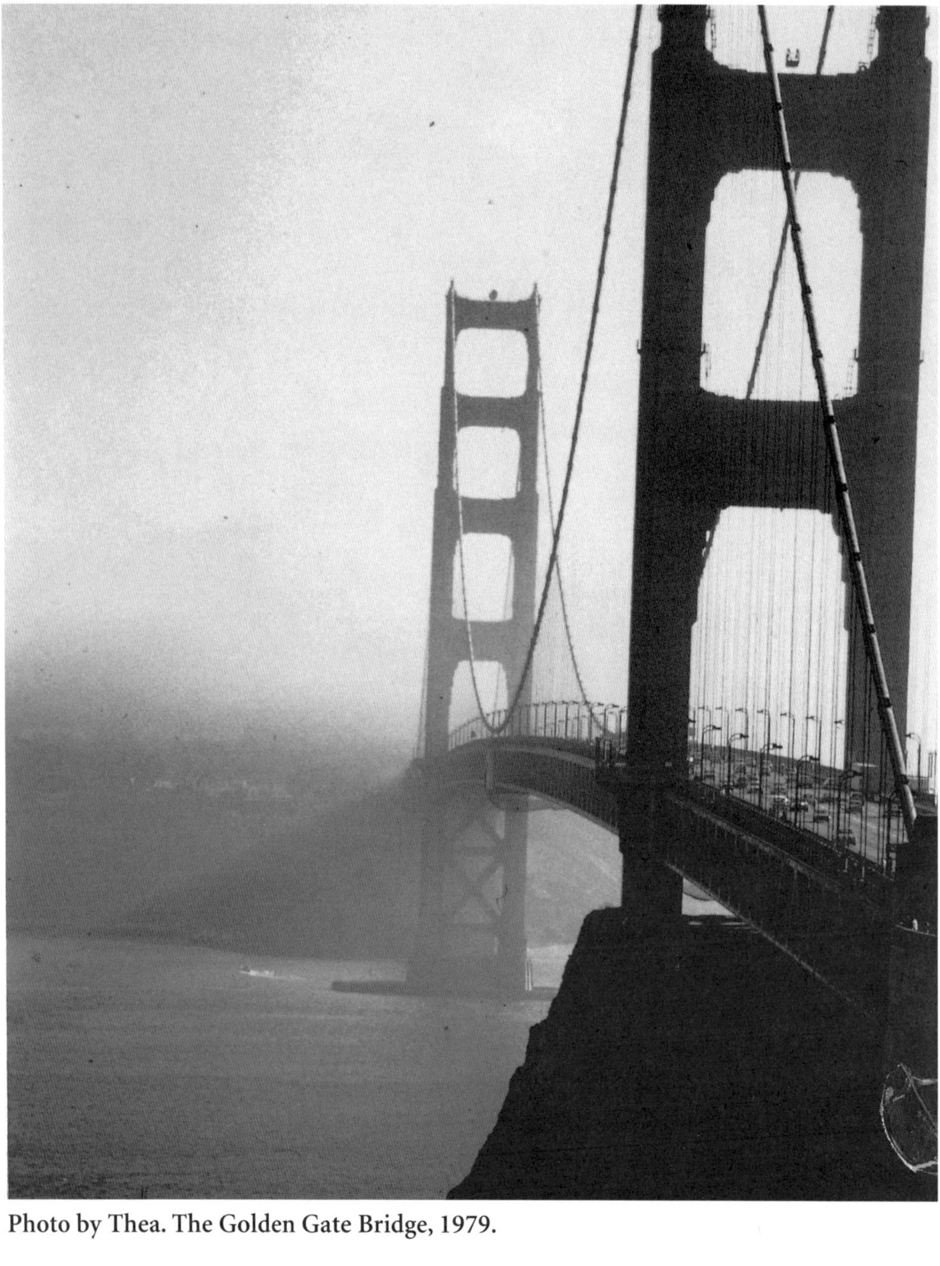

Photo by Thea. The Golden Gate Bridge, 1979.

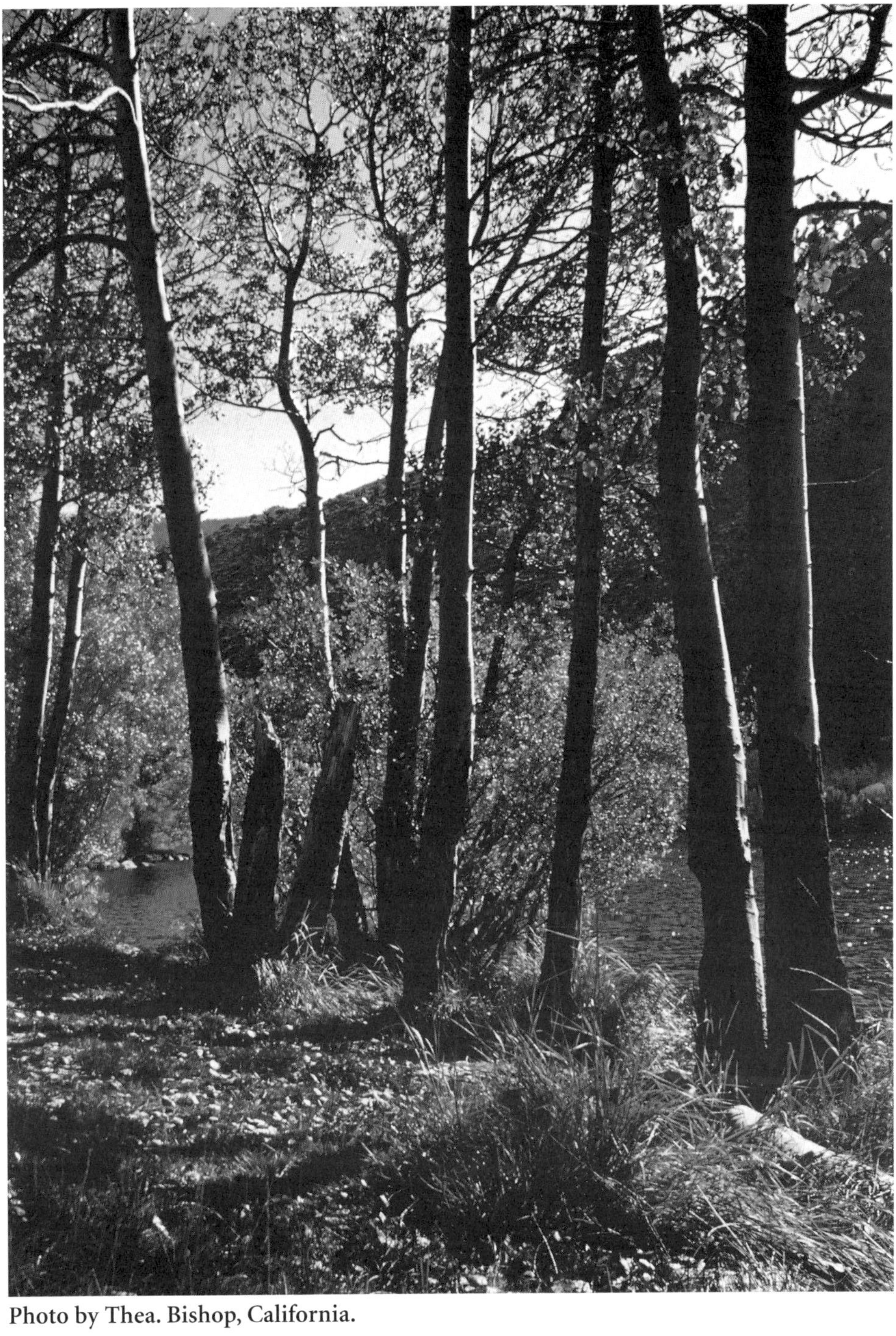

Photo by Thea. Bishop, California.

Disclaimer

The following list of suggested supplements and other items is simply that—a suggestion. I do hope that the ones I have selected will give you more insight into what is available and may be helpful to you. Proper nutrition is so important. Remember, as time passes, treatments for illnesses change. The following suggestions are only a partial listing of what may be available. Please do not rush to the health food store after reading this section. As I am not a nutritionist yet, please discuss these suggestions with your healthcare provider to see what will work best for you. Correct dosage combination is of **utmost** importance.

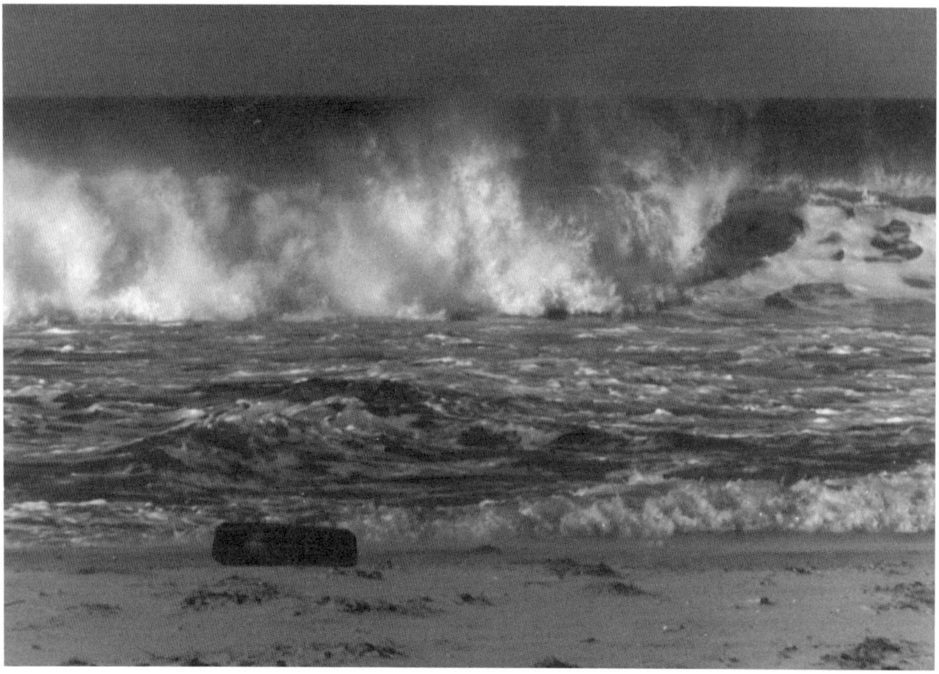

Photo by Thea.

Chapter Six

Suggested Supplements and Good Nutrition

Vitamin B-Complex

The B-complex vitamins are essential for normal functioning of the nervous system. In fact, they are most likely the most important vitamins for a healthy nervous system. Because they are water soluble and any excess in our body is quickly excreted, they must be continuously replaced for optimum health.

B12—Sublingual

Vitamin B12 is highly respected for its energy-giving properties. However, much of its benefits occur in the digestive tract. Besides by injection, B12 can be taken sublingually, which is the most effective way for it to be taken. It is important to use a formula that also has folic acid. Lately, I have been taking 2cc of vitamin B12 intramuscularly once a week and B12 with folic acid sublingually after breakfast. By now, I have had so many shots that I truly welcome the B12 sublingually.

Chromium GTF

Most of us with CFIDS have hypoglycemia. Research is showing that chromium can be very effective in helping to control low blood sugar, build muscle, burn fat, and give energy.

Chromium is an important trace mineral that is necessary for our key metabolic hormone to do its job of maintaining healthy blood sugar levels. Studies have shown that ninety percent of Americans are

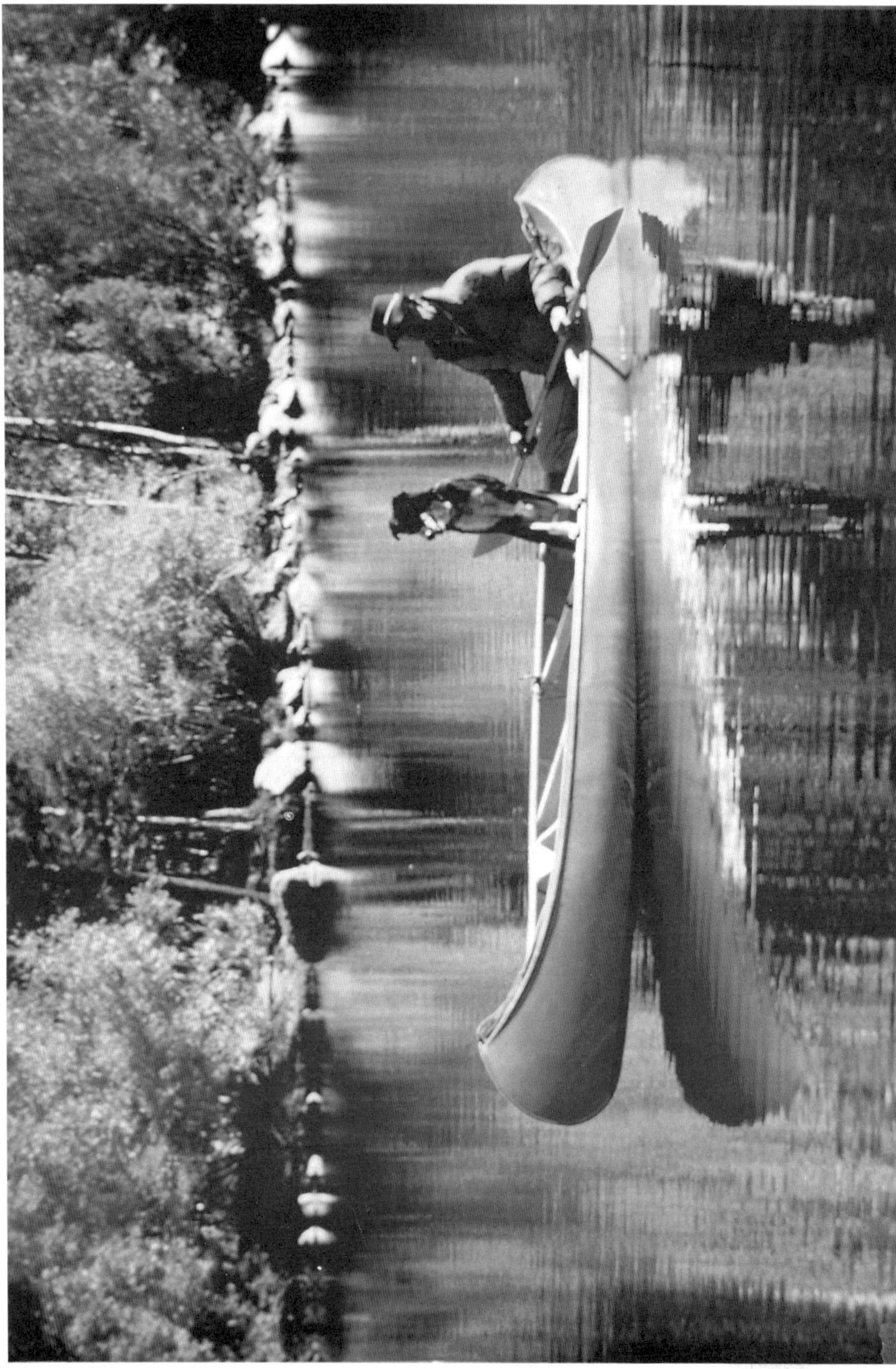

Photo by Thea. Bishop, CA, 1983. Photography trip with Karl.

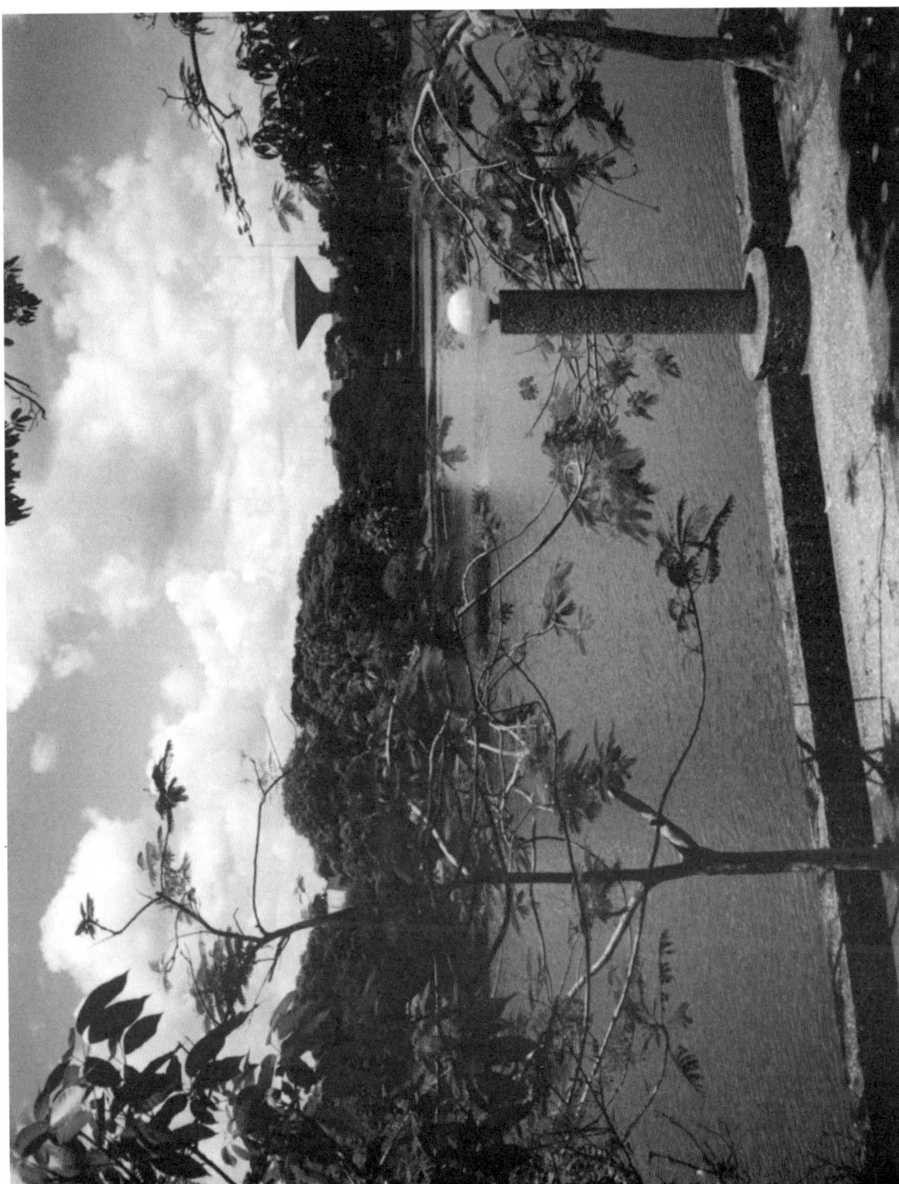

Photo by Thea. Tabasco, Mexico, 1995.

chromium-deficient! Chromium usually comes in 200 mg tablets. The GTF stands for glucose tolerance factor.

Vitamin B6

Vitamin B6 is involved in more body functions than any other single nutrient. Vitamin B6 has an effect on both physical and mental health. Vitamin B6, or pyridoxine, is necessary for the absorption of fats and the production of hydrochloric acid, which are responsible for maintaining a sodium and potassium balance and promoting red blood cell formation. The nervous system depends on vitamin B6 to help the brain synthesize DNA and RNA.

Research has shown that too much B6 can promote nerve damage.

Zinc

Zinc is an essential trace mineral, crucial in the absorption process of vitamins and a constituent of at least twenty-five enzymes involved in digestion and metabolism. Zinc plays a crucial role in the absorption process of the B-complex vitamins and carbonic anhydrase, which is necessary for tissue respiration. Usually 50 mg of zinc daily will help prevent zinc deficiency.

Evening Primrose Oil

Evening primrose oil contains linoceid acid and gamma linolec acid C-glad. These are two very important polyunsaturated fatty acids, which are necessary for the proper metabolism in cells. Like vitamins, essential fatty acids (EFAs) must be of primary consideration in your diet, because the body is unable to manufacture them. Evening primrose oil produces prostaglandin, which is necessary for the health of all cells. EFAs are also used by your body to provide energy, maintain body temperature, insulate the nerves, and protect the tissues.

Garlic

Garlic has been used for its healing qualities for more than 5,000 years. It has been reported to be one of the world's oldest natural remedies known to man. Garlic can help boost the immune system, as well as support the cardiovascular, circulatory, and respiratory systems. It fights infection, aids in the digestion process, and has been found to be beneficial for lowering cholesterol.

Milk Thistle

Milk thistle is a potent liver-cleansing herb. It can protect and restore the liver compound, silymarin, found naturally in the seeds and flowers of the milk thistle plant. Sylimarin has been shown to help the liver fight off toxins and pollutants, produce new liver cells, and prevent cellular damage.

Malic Acid

This is also a very important supplement. It helps reduce muscle pain and fatigue. According to an article I read recently, about 40% of CFIDS survivors benefit from malic acid.

Fresh Juices

Not only are fruit and vegetable juices your best convenience foods, but they also provide thousands of beneficial substances, some with well-known functions and some whose role in the human body are not yet understood or recognized.

Fruits and vegetables contain substantial amounts of carbohydrates, which supply most of the energy we use to live and perform work. Fruits and vegetables also contain many amounts of vitamins that regulate the metabolism and help convert fats and carbohydrates into energy. They also contain minerals that are necessary for nerve and muscle function and are a necessary building material for some body tissue.

Fruit and vegetable juices have protective effects that can prevent major diseases like cancer and heart attacks. Many vegetables and fruits are high in substances called antioxidants such as beta carotene, vitamin C, vitamin E, and the mineral selenium. All of these protect cell membranes from damage caused by free radicals.

Fruits and vegetables can be our best non-prescription drug. For example, ginger is well recognized as a cure for motion sickness and nausea. Cabbage juice is good for healing stomach ulcers. Cranberry juice is wonderful for urinary tract infections, which are so common among CFIDS patients.

Fresh juices are a perfect food supplement. Personally, at times, I do not have the energy to make fresh juice from scratch. So I usually buy frozen fruits and vegetables and put them in the blender. You can also put them through a juicer if you have one! I like adding garlic, cayenne pepper, and sometimes I'll even add a quarter of an avocado. Experiment to see what delicious and healthy combinations you can come up with!

Fresh juices are extremely important in rebuilding a weakened immune system. One glass of carrot juice, for example, with celery or broccoli juice is a powerful antioxidant drink as it is full of vitamins A and C, as well as a vast array of other vitamins and minerals.

I prefer to dilute my fresh juices, because I have hypoglycemia and Candida, both of which are sensitive to the high sugar content in fresh fruit and vegetable juices. Also, if you've never experienced fresh juice, you may want to begin with half water and half juice. As always, it is best to get advice from your health-care provider when doing anything new.

It is definitely well worth the effort, and I know it is an effort, to treat yourself to a fresh vegetable or fruit juice.

Pycnogenol

The extraordinary antioxidant properties of pycnogenol are attributed to the fact that it is not a single bioflavonoid, but a complex combination of bioflavonoids. Pycnogenol has an exceptionally high level of proanthocyanidins (the main active ingredient), and it also contains other water-soluble bioflavinoids. This unique combination provides a powerful, completely balanced, all-natural antioxidant.

Pycnogenol is found only in non-chemically processed maritime pine bark. It usually comes in 20 mg tablets or capsules. The recommended intake is 20 mg (one capsule or tablet) for every twenty pounds of body weight.

Colloidal Silver

Colloidal silver has been around since the late 1800s and has been recognized by the FDA as having therapeutic value. Silver is a natural antibiotic that in a colloidal state, kills every harmful bacterium and virus with which it comes in contact. All bacteria, virus, and fungus organisms are killed within six minutes of contact.

One might ask, "How do we get silver in our bodies in the first place?" We get silver and all minerals into the body through the food we eat. How does silver get in the food? Through living soil. Billions of organisms can be found in a handful of soil. These living organisms break down the soil into minerals in a form amiable to the plant. When we eat these plants, the minerals are transferred to the digestive tract, where our bodies distribute the captured organic chelated minerals through the bloodstream to various organs of the body. Hence, we get silver from plants. Some people cannot assimilate silver for some reason, or as the tissues age, we develop a silver deficiency and an impaired immune system.

Colloidal silver is the only known substance that can safely be used as a silver supplement. A teaspoon a day is the recommended dosage. It has also been recommended to me by Dr. Roy Kupsinel to be taken intravenously, although, I have not tried it yet.

Blue-Green Algae

This product is one of the most powerful and complete food supplements available on the market today. Steven Boehm, Vice President of the Chronic Fatigue Media Awareness Association and President of Efficient Systems, is a supplier of this remarkable product.

Water

The human body is composed of approximately seventy percent water. Water is involved in nearly every body process, including digestion, absorption, circulation, and excretion. Water is also the primary transporter of nutrients throughout the body and is necessary for all building functions in the body. The body cannot survive without water for longer than five days. Personally, I drink distilled water. I also invested in a water filter, but I still get the taste from tap water. Now, there are many types of drinking water. For example, mineral water, fluoridated water, and natural spring water. You need to be the judge of which is best for you or talk to your health-care provider.

They may be able to explain what would be the best water for you to consume.

Drinking at least eight glasses of water a day is recommended. I often add lemon to the water, which is also beneficial for detoxification.

Vitamin C

Vitamin C does many things. For example, it is a powerful antioxidant, helps the nervous system, is an immune enhancer, fights colds and flu, and can help prevent many illnesses.

Vitamin A and Beta Carotene

Vitamin A is stored in the liver; therefore, you can only take it for a short time if you take a lot. Taking beta carotene is different. Beta carotene is safe, even in higher amounts. It works as an antioxidant to defend against the damaging activity of oxidized free radicals that are dangerous to healthy tissues.

Vitamin/Mineral Formula

Again, a good vitamin/mineral formula is advisable. There are many brands on the market. Personally, I buy many supplements from the CFIDS Buyer's Club and Kaisers Nutrition Center in Santa Barbara. The body needs more than seventy minerals to maintain good health. Often, we do not absorb mineral formulas in tablet form. I suggest trying liquid mineral supplements, which are absorbed by the body at a rate of about ninety percent. Minerals activate more than three hundred enzymes and are crucial to the production and release of energy.

Coenzyme Q10

Many physicians recommend this supplement. Among them are Jay Goldstein, M.D., Henry Hoegerman, M.D., Paul Chenney, M.D., and Daniel Peterson, M.D. They have all found that about half of the patients treated will experience reduced pain, fatigue, and exercise intolerance, as well as an increase in stamina, with little to no adverse reaction. There have been entire books dedicated to the fantastic effectiveness of coenzyme Q10.

Calcium and Magnesium

A good balanced formula is extremely important. Calcium and magnesium are important for better bone formation, as well as for the nervous system and muscles. Symptoms of calcium and magnesium deficiency include feeling tired, insomnia, muscle twitches, and brittle nails. Take as recommended for best results.

Melatonin

This seems to be the hottest thing in sleeping pills. It's natural, it's cheap, and it works. Can it really be that good? Many people find that it works extremely well. Personally, I cannot take it because it makes me ill.

We produce melatonin abundantly throughout early life. Then, right before puberty, the level of melatonin in the blood drops slightly, continuing to decline steadily into old age. Melatonin is a hormone produced by the pineal gland. Research suggests that it could boost your immune system, combat jet lag, protect cells from free radical damage, prevent cancer, and extend life!

For now, consumers are stuck deciding whether to trust what they read on a label. Dr. Paul Lisson and his colleagues in Monza, Italy, did extensive research on melatonin. For more information, go to your favorite health food store or book store. I hope you have better luck with melatonin than I have. I will probably try to take it again in doses of 1/2 to 1 mg. As with all of the supplements described in this book, each of us must test individually to see what works and does not work.

Essential Fatty Acids

There are two essential fatty acids. These essential nutrients have been shown by leading researchers to be necessary for both the optimum health of the body and freedom from degenerative disease. They are known as omega 3 (alpha-linolic acid or ALNA) and omega 6 (linolic acid or LA).

Along with protein, essential fatty acids are the building blocks of cell membranes and various internal cell structures.

Essential fatty acids are necessary for:

- metabolism and transportation of triglycerides and cholesterol.
- development and function of the human brain.
- proper function of vision, nervous system, adrenal glands, and testes, playing a vital role in sperm formation and conception.
- boosting metabolism, metabolic rate, energy production, and oxygen uptake.

Essential fatty acids, particularly omega 3, have been shown to decrease the growth of cancer cells, Candida, and various anaerobic organisms destructive to the health of the body.

Amino Acids

Each amino acid has specific functions and is needed to prevent various symptoms from developing. The many functions and deficiency symptoms of twenty-eight amino acids are described in most nutritional and vitamin books. I would like to outline some of the amino acid family, which may be the most important with CFIDS survivors.

L-Taurine

L-taurine is an essential amino aid found in high concentrations in the heart muscle, white blood cells, skeletal muscle, and central nervous system. This amino acid aids in fat digestion, heart disorders, hypoglycemia, orthorosclerosis, hypertension, and edema and acts as a building block for all amino acids. It is a key component of bile, which is needed for the digestion of fats, absorption of fat soluble vitamins, and control of serum and cholesterol levels. Epilepsy, anxiety, hyperactivity, and poor brain function are all related to the deficiency of L-taurine. However, L-taurine is NOT found in most animal proteins. Therefore, synthesis in the body is CRUCIAL. Taurine may be synthesized from cysteine, but it requires vitamin B6 for this conversion.

L-Glutamine

L-glutamine is known to be fuel for the brain. This amino acid is very dominant in cerebrospinal fluid, and many people claim that it is useful in alleviating depression, reducing fatigue, improving memory and other cognitive functions, and reducing sugar and simple carbohydrate cravings. I usually take a complex amino acid formula and add L-glutamine, as well as L-lysine, another useful amino acid, when I first wake up, on an empty stomach or at least two hours after a meal. I have been advised to not take L-glutamine, because it could trigger a seizure and, as I have mentioned earlier, I have a seizure disorder.

L-Tyrosine

L-tyrosine is very important in the treatment of anxiety, depression, allergies, and headaches. It aids in the production of melanin (pigment of the skin and hair) and in the function of the adrenal, thyroid, and pituitary glands. L-tyrosine is also used to synthesize epinephrine and dopamine. It has been used successfully to aid in the withdrawal from drugs.

DL-Phenylanine

DL-phenylanine is very effective in the control of pain, especially for those with arthritis. It functions as a building block of all amino acids, increases mental alertness, suppresses the appetite, and aids in the treatment of Parkinson's disease. Use DL-phenylanine with caution if you are pregnant, diabetic or have high blood pressure.

L-Lysine

L-lysine is an essential building block for all protein. It is needed for proper bone development in children and helps in calcium absorption. It also maintains nitrogen balance in adults. Among the many functions of this amino acids are its ability to fight cold sores and Herpes viruses; aid in the production of antibodies, hormones, and enzymes; help in collagen formation; and help in the repair of tissue. L-lysine deficiency results in loss of energy, inability to concentrate, irritability, bloodshot eyes, hair loss, anemia, retarded growth, and reproduction disorder.

L-Phenylalanine

L-phenylalanine is often used to treat depression. It produces neurotransmitters; is used by the brain to manufacture norepinephrine; and aids in memory, learning, and dealing with obesity. Because of its action in the central nervous system, this amino acid elevates moods; enables the individual to overcome depression; and decreases the pain associated with migraines, PMS, and arthritis. Do not take L-phenylalanine if you are pregnant, have high blood pressure, or have pre-existing pigmented melanoma (a type of cancer).

A Listing of Foods and Their Benefits

MAGNESIUM
Rye (whole)
Oranges
Lemons
Grapefruit
Chives
Onions
Sea-Fish

CHLORINE
Watercress
Dill
Kale
Goat Cheese
Asparagus
Sea-Fish
Eggplant
Red Meat
Cow's Milk
Coconuts
Sweet Potatoes
Pineapple
Cottage Cheese
Whole Wheat Bread
Turnips
Whey
Tomatoes
Carrots
Parsnips
Cabbage
Cucumbers
Spinach
Celery
Beets
Swiss Chard
Lettuce
Egg Whites
Butter

SODIUM
Pumpkin
Rutabaga
Dill
Celery
Romaine
Turnips
Gizzards
Buttermilk
Pistachio Nuts
Bananas
Black Figs
Ox Joints
Cucumbers
Asparagus
Swiss Chard
Whey
Beets
Avocado
Spinach
Cabbage
Butter
Roquefort Cheese
Pumpernickel
Goat Cheese
Radishes
Leeks
Okra
Gelatin
Watercress
Eggs
Pomegranates
Carrots

A Listing of Foods and Their Benefits

Apples
Tomatoes
Strawberries
Lettuce
Dandelion

FLUORINE
Mackerel
Oxtail Broth
Cod Liver Oil
Swiss Cheese
Gelatin
Goat's Milk
Oysters
Roquefort Cheese

SILICON
Cabbage
Onions
Leeks
Cherries
Rice
Parsnips
Artichokes
Apricots
Strawberries
Goat Cheese
Rhubarb
Dandelion
Whole Oats
Figs
Horseradish
Lettuce
Asparagus
Cucumbers
Pumpkin
Beets
Spinach

MANGANESE
Romaine
Chestnuts
Peppermint
Liver
Almonds
Dill
Pignolia Nuts
Walnuts
Parsley

IODINE
All Seafood
Kelp
Onions
Grapes
Turnips
Salmon
Potato Skins
Tomatoes
Dulse
Green Peas
Oysters
Artichokes
Pineapple
Natural Rice

IRON
Cherries
Celery
Cabbage
Beef
Strawberries
Raisins
Tomatoes
Carrots
Spinach
Artichokes
Black Figs
Mushrooms
Prunes
Asparagus
Leeks
Watermelon
Turnips
Dill
Potato Skins
Liver
Lettuce
Oysters
Romaine
Kale
Onions
Radishes
Bone Marrow
Sorrel
Gooseberries
Cauliflower
Kohlrabi
Cucumbers
Horseradish
Rhubarb
Rice
Swiss Chard
Dandelion
Rutabaga

A Listing of Foods and Their Benefits

Pumpkin
Parsley
Beets

CALCIUM
Celery
Carrots
Cucumbers
Peas
Turnips
Dandelion
Tomatoes
Beechnut
String Beans
Romaine
Chives
Dates
Sea-Fish
Leek Leaf
Dill
Turnips
Onions
Watercress
Pumpkin
Orange
Strawberries
Cranberries
Blackberries
Cabbage
Okra
Kale
Asparagus
Radishes
Spinach
Goat's Milk
Cow's Milk
Buttermilk
Skim Milk
Lettuce
Rhubarb
Swiss Chard
Whole Grains
Lemons
Cottage Cheese

SULFUR
Radishes
Mustard Greens
String Beans
Green Peas
Turnips
Brussels Sprouts
Spinach
Garlic
Cucumbers
Cabbage
Watercress
Cauliflower
Parsnip
Tomatoes
Sorrel
Kale
Onions
Cranberries
Raspberries
Lettuce
Figs
Egg Yolk
Dill
Chives

POTASSIUM
Mushrooms
Cucumbers
Onions
Turnips
Dill
Sweet Potatoes
Soya Beans
Lima Beans
Celery
Tomatoes
Asparagus
Eggplant
Brussels Sprouts
Kidney Beans
Kale
Watercress
Bitter Herbs
String Beans
Potato Skins
Artichokes
Radishes
Cabbage
Cherries
Apricots
Watermelon
Grapes
Lemons
Limes
Peaches
Prunes
Huckleberries
Rhubarb
Parsnips
Rutabaga

A Listing of Foods and Their Benefits

Sorrel
Spinach
Molasses
Kohlrabi
Leek Leaf
Dandelion
Beets
Carrots
Lettuce
Cauliflower
Swiss Chard
Skim Milk

MAGNESIUM
Apples
Tomatoes
Beets
Dill
Rutabaga
Whole Barley
Watercress
Wheat Germ
Chick Peas
Cabbage
Blackberries
Whole Oats
Lettuce
Sorrel
Kale
Turnips
Dandelion
Spinach
Romaine
Rice
Kohlrabi
Almonds
Celery
Swiss Chard

PHOSPHOROUS
Whole Wheat
Romaine
Whole Oats
Rice
Spinach
Turnips
Egg Yolks
Mushrooms
Currants
Kale
Soya Beans
Asparagus
Sorrel
Celery
Buttermilk
Radishes
Rhubarb
Peas
Whole Barley
Fish
Dill
Wheat Bran
Almonds
Walnuts
Lettuce
Cucumbers
Brussels Sprouts
Cottage Cheese
Cauliflower
Pumpkin
Beans
Cabbage
Swiss Chard
Goat's Milk

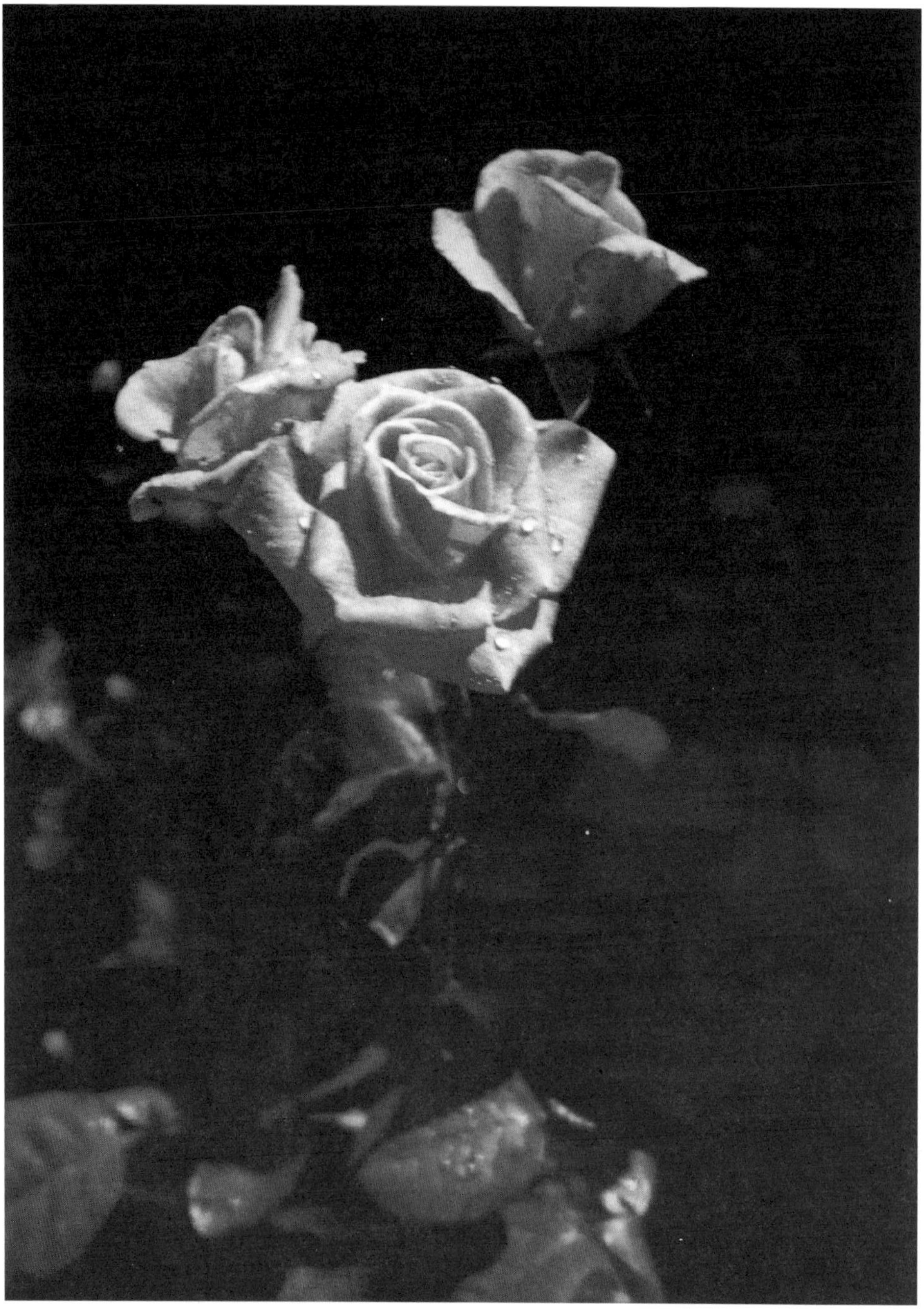

Photo by Thea. "The Beauty of a Rose."

Selected Inspirational Poems and Quotes

If I can stop one heart from breaking,
I shall not live in vain:
If I can ease one life the aching,
Or cool one pain,
Or help one fainting robin
Unto his nest again,
I shall not live in vain.

Emily Dickinson

My personal reflection: Quite frankly, and with innermost honesty to you, the reader, this poem brought tears to my eyes. I started this book with the simple desire that I would be able to help at least one other CFIDS survivor, in hopes that they would not have to go through what I experienced before finally being correctly diagnosed. "Not in vain," reminded me of sitting for countless hours, day or night, whenever I had the energy, writing down experiences, feelings, and ideas. The creation of "Beyond The Dark Cloud," was indeed, "not in vain."

Abide the hour, for all
Is but a passing thing;
And should the heaven's fall,
A lark will Earthward wing.

Johann Wolfgang Von Goethe

ꕥ

Do thou but hold thy peace and wait
Though round thee storms be blowing:
And conscious thus of mortal fate,
More God-like wilt be growing.

Johann Wolfgang Von Goethe

ꕥ

God grant me the serenity
to accept the things I cannot change,
The courage to change the things I can
And the knowledge to know the difference.

Author unknown

My personal reflection: With an illness such as CFIDS, I think and feel that all we can do is accept this mysterious illness and make the best of it. We need all of our wisdom, guiding us to faith and inner strength every second of the day. All of us CFIDS survivors have the courage to that; we just need to accept this illness with grace and determination.

ꕥ

The Daffodils

I wandered lonely as a cloud
That floats on high o'er vales and hills,
When all at once I saw a crowd,
A host, of golden daffodils;
Beside the lake, beneath the trees,
Fluttering and dancing in the breeze.

Continuous as the stars that shine
And twinkle on the milky way,
They stretched in never-ending line
Along the margin of a bay;
Ten thousand saw I at a glance,
Tossing their heads in sprightly dance.

The waves beside them danced; but they
Outdid the sparkling waves in glee;
A poet could not but be gay,
In such a jocund company:
I gazed—and gazed—but little thought
What wealth the show to me had brought.

For oft, when on my couch I lie
In vacant or in pensive mood,
They flash upon that inward eye
Which is the bliss of solitude;
And then my heart with pleasure fills,
And dances with the daffodils.

William Wordsworth

In matters of principle, stand like a rock.
In matters of taste, swim with the current.
Thomas Jefferson

My personal reflection: All we can do
as we endure is swim with the current
and stand like a rock.

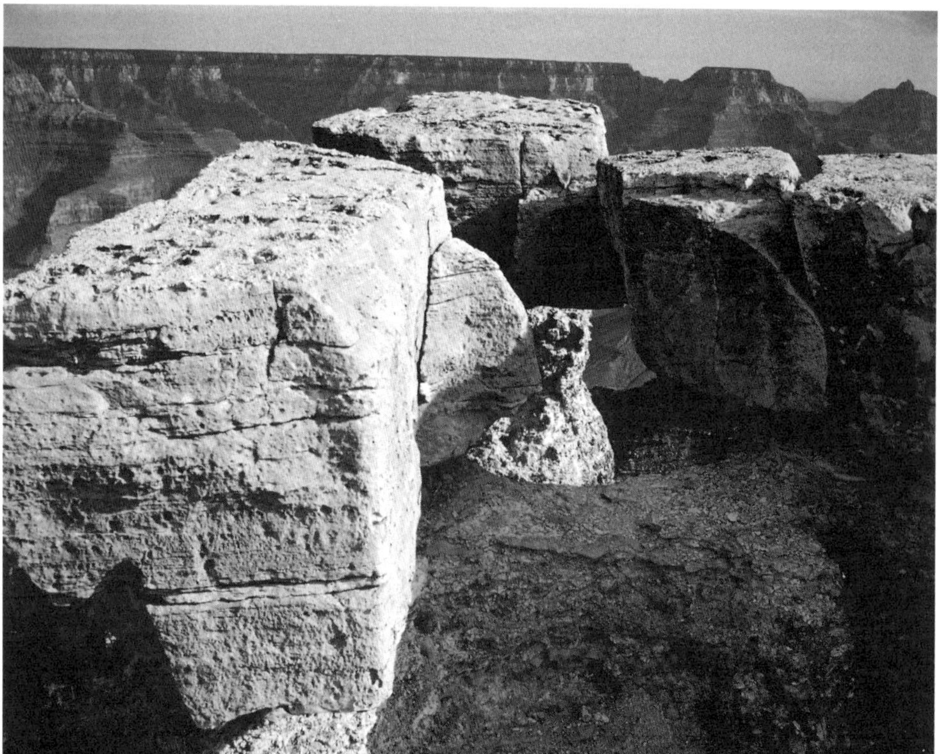

Photo by Thea. Grand Canyon, 1983.

Comes the Dawn

After a while you learn the subtle difference
Between holding a hand and chaining a soul,
And you learn that love doesn't mean security,
And you begin to learn that kisses aren't contracts
And presents aren't promises,
And you begin to accept your defeats
With your head up and your eyes down
With the grace of a woman, not the grief of a child,
And learn to build all your roads
On today because tomorrow's ground
Is too uncertain for plans, and futures have
A way of falling down in mid-flight.
After a while you learn that even sunshine
Burns if you get too much.
So you plant your own garden and decorate
Your own soul, instead of waiting
For someone to bring you flowers.
And you learn that you really can endure...
That you really are strong
And you really do have worth.
And you learn and learn...
With every good-bye, you learn.

Author unknown

Life is a series of collisions with
the future;
It is not the sum of what we have been,
but what we yearn to be.

José Ortega y Gasset (1883-1955)

My personal reflection: CFIDS brings us to collisions in life that we never thought would happen to us. It is such a total body disease. But out of this challenge, we can become better people, and the challenge to fight this disease is a part of the collisions with our future that we can master with hard work, God's help, and most of all, our own inner strength, which we all have. Then we can taste again what life used to be.

Man is what he believes.

Anton Chekov (1860-1904)

My personal reflection: If you believe you'll get better, then most likely it will come true.

Success is never final and failure never fatal.
It's courage that counts!

Successful unlimited

My personal reflection: In a sense, CFIDS survivors are very successful because we have the endurance to cope with CFIDS, as well as the courage to survive in spite of the many obstacles we encounter.

To be upset over what you
don't have is to waste what you
do have.

Ken S. Keys, Jr.

My personal reflection: This principle goes for all of us who endure CFIDS. I do feel that we are responsible for our own lives, and we must seek every avenue to make ourselves feel better. Some of you can only stay in bed all the time. I know how it feels, I've been there, but we can say to ourselves, regardless of how we feel, "Thank you God for another day, and thank you God for helping me find the road to recovery." Regardless of your circumstances, you will then begin to feel better, and better, and better. Enough now, back to bed and rest, listen to the music and the birds outside. No...this is not a wasted day at all.

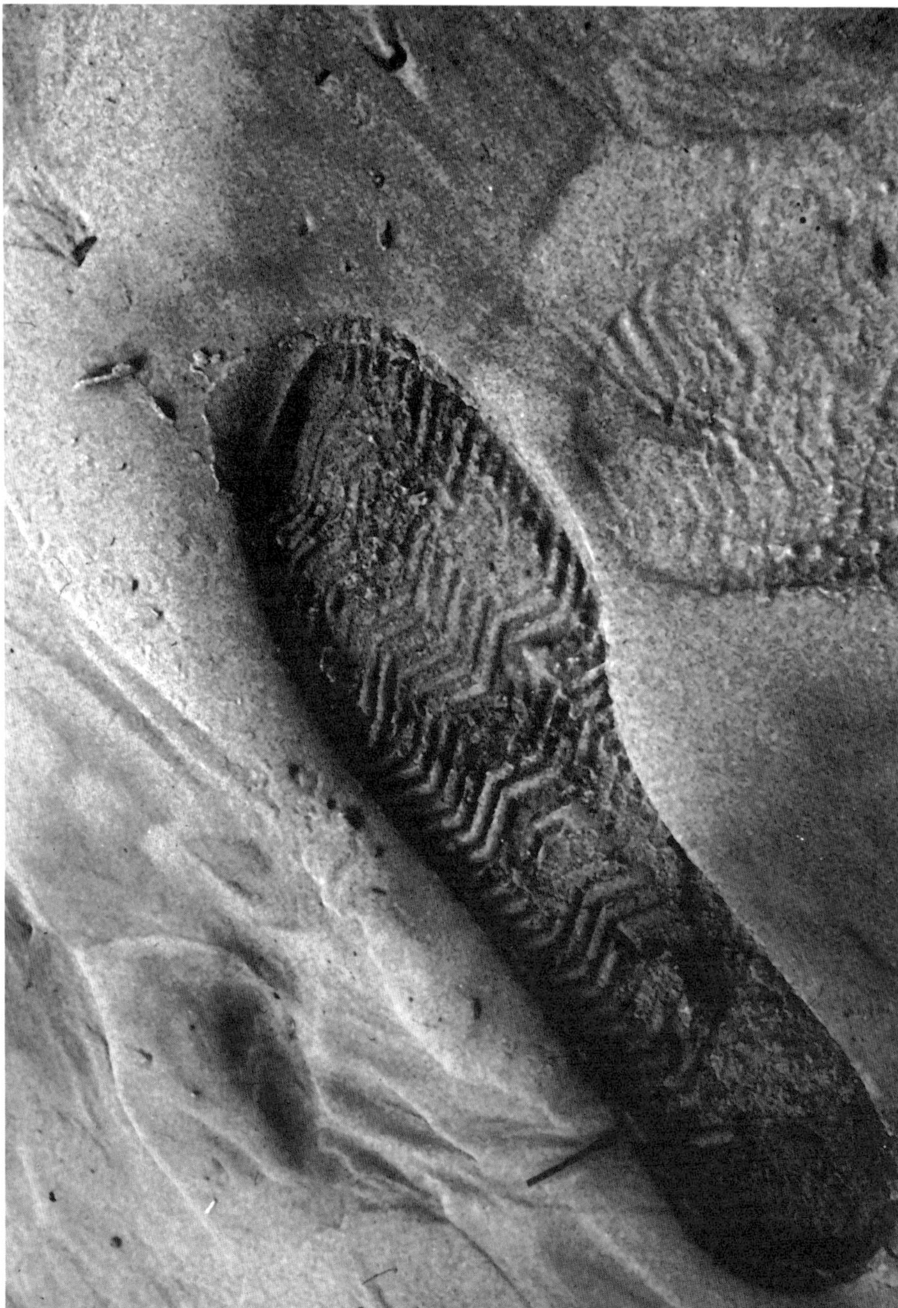

Photo by Thea. My footprints in the sand of a beach in Southern California.

Footprints

One night a man had a dream. He dreamed that he was walking along the beach with the Lord. Across the sky flashed scenes from his life. For each scene, he noticed two sets of footprints in the sand. One belonged to him, and the other to the Lord.

When the last scene of his life flashed before him, he looked back at the footprints in the sand. He noticed that many times along the path of his life there was only one set of footprints. He also noticed that it happened at the very lowest and saddest times in his life.

This really bothered him and he questioned the Lord about it: "Lord, you said that once I decided to follow you, you'd walk with me all the way. But I have noticed that during the most troublesome times in my life, there is only one set of footprints. I don't understand why when I needed you, you would leave me."

The Lord replied, "My precious, precious child, I love you and I would never leave you. During your times of trial and suffering, when you see only one set of footprints, it was then that I carried you."

The will to win is not nearly as important
as the will to prepare to win.

Bobby Knight

My personal reflection: Quite frankly, this monstrous disease is a challenge every second of every day. I want to win this battle—and win I will! Whatever it takes, I want to get back to good health. Yes, I feel defeated at times or perhaps often, but not for long. I think of what I have, that is life, and where there is life, there is hope. Because I was the champion swimmer, I was given the historic honor of representing the town of Voitzberg on its 700th-year birthday in 1949. I had to prepare hard to win this fantastic event, but it was well worth it.

(See photo below.)

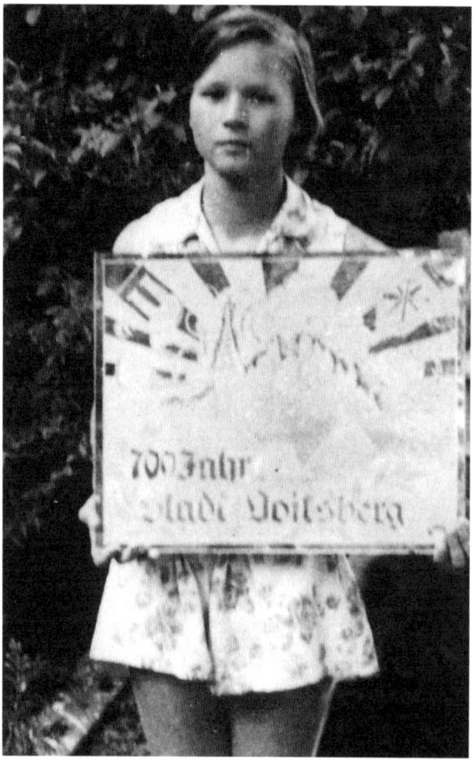

Thea Hermesmeyer, my maiden name.

Dreams are the touchstones of our characters.

Henry David Thoreau (1817-1862)

My personal reflection: Without dreams, we could easily stop taking advantage of what God has given us freely. Before going to bed, select what you want to dream about, make it positive, regardless of the circumstances. The reward will be that your dreams will eventually turn into reality.

The worst prison would be a closed heart.

Pope John Paul II

My personal reflection: When we are in pain and ill, we often close our eyes and hearts. It is only human to do so. I do that, but quickly remind myself not to. It would only lead to defeat and worsen my condition. Let us try to keep our eyes and hearts open with love and understanding for each other and ourselves. Let us love God, who gave us this life. Having CFIDS often feels overwhelming, and we feel like prisoners, trapped by this diabolical disease. Keep in mind that love is the most powerful healer in the universe.

There are two days we should never worry about.
Yesterday: With its heartaches and mistakes.
They are gone forever

Tomorrow: Is the other day.
It has problems and possibilities, but until the sun rises,
it is unborn and unreal.

Today: Today is the only day that matters.
Only when we add the burdens of those other days
are we likely to fail.

Author unknown

My personal reflection: If we can make today count to its fullest, regardless of how we feel about other days, tomorrow will be better.

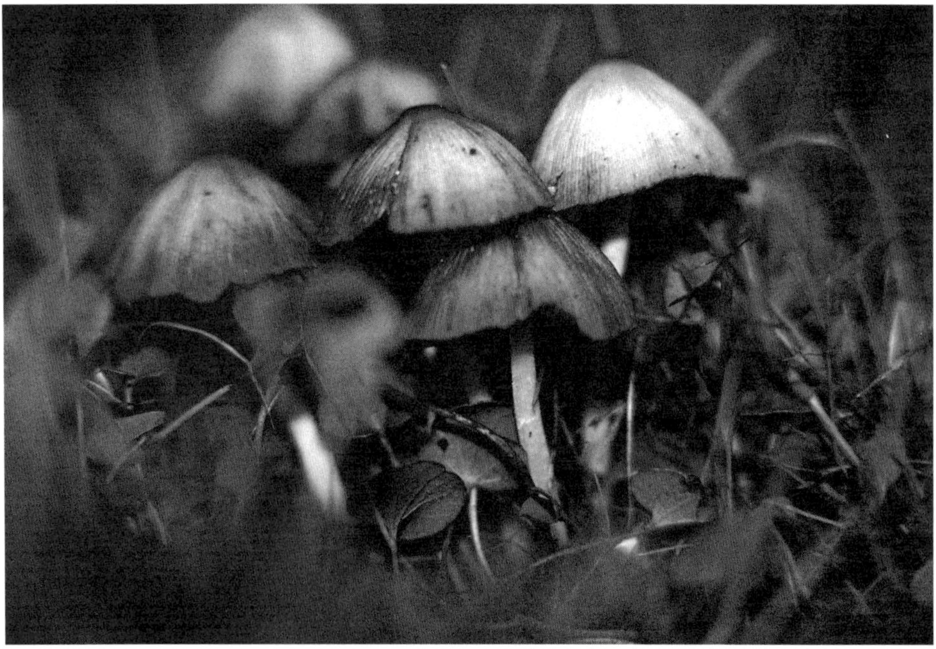

Photo by Thea.

Waiting

Serene, I fold my hands and wait,
Nor care for wind nor tide nor sea;
I rave no more 'gainst time or fate,
For lo! my own shall come to me.

I stay my haste, I make delays—
For what avails this eager pace?
I stand amid the eternal ways
And what is mine shall know my face.

Asleep, awake, by night or day,
The friends I seek are seeking me,
No wind can drive my bark astray
Nor change the tide of destiny.

What matter if I stand alone?
I wait with joy the coming years;
My heart shall reap where it has sown,
And garner up its fruit of tears.

The waters know their own, and draw
The brook that springs in yonder height;
So flows the good with equal law
Unto the soul of pure delight.

The stars come nightly to the sky;
The tidal wave unto the sea;
Nor time, nor space, nor deep, nor high,
Can keep my own away from me.

John Burroughs

Be Strong

Be strong!
We are not here to play, to dream, to drift;
We have hard work to do, and loads to lift;
Shun not the struggle—face it; 'tis God's gift.

Be strong!
Say not, "The days are evil. Who's to blame?"
And fold the hands and acquiesce—oh shame!
Stand up, speak out, and bravely, in God's name.

Be strong!
It matters not how deep intrenched the wrong,
How hard the battle goes, the day how long;
Faint not—fight on! Tomorrow comes the song.

Maltbie Davenport Babcock

If we never lose anything, we will never know how much we once had.

Thea Schlosser

My personal reflection: At times, life offers us a lot, but we are not able to appreciate it and often take things for granted. Then something bad happens. That is when we realize the most what we once had

Broken Dreams

As children bring their broken toys
With tears for us to mend.
I brought my broken dreams to God
Because He was my friend.
But then instead of leaving Him
in peace to work alone,
I hung around and tried to help
With ways that were my own.
At last I snatched them back and cried,
"How can you be so slow"—
"My child," He said,
"What could I do?
You never did let go."

Author unknown

My personal reflection: Having CFIDS is not a
broken dream, it is a new beginning,
love and compassion, Thea.

Ever mounting higher, higher
Ever further I must gaze!

Johann Wolfgang Von Goethe

Remember that all you possess in the world will be found, at the moment of your death, to belong to someone else, but all that you are will be yours forever.

Author unknown

My personal reflection: No matter how rich we are in material things, it is how rich we are in our hearts and souls that defines us. Unfortunately, money is a necessity in order to survive in this society; however, I truly believe that what we do for others will be responsible for most of our happiness.

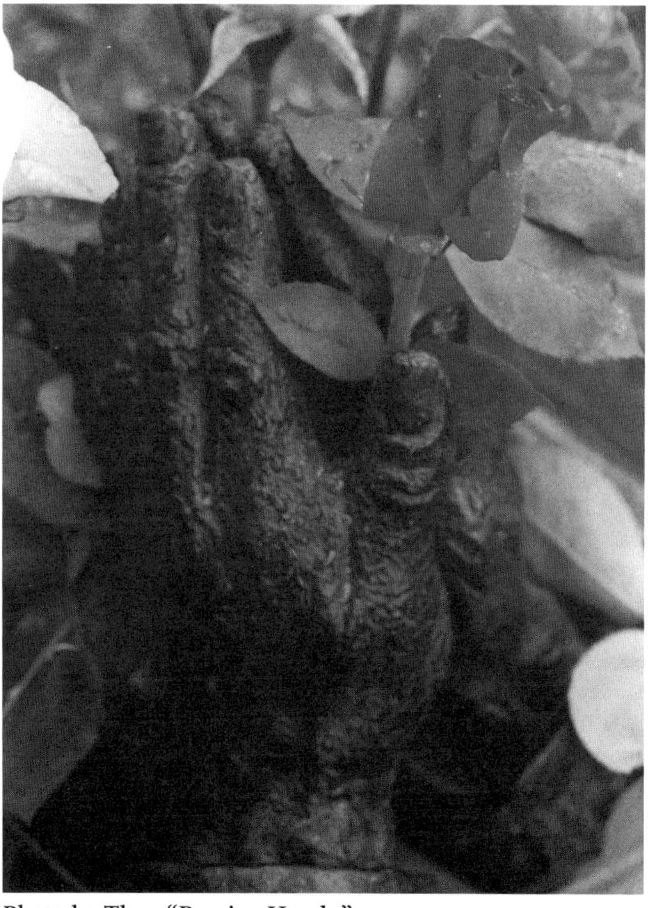

Photo by Thea. "Praying Hands."

And in today—already walks tomorrow.
Samuel Taylor Coleridge (1772-1834)

My personal reflection: Can you see from this beautiful thought how important it is to plant ideas, hopes, and dreams? This is our life. Yes, we are ill, but let's never forget to plant that seed of positive thought, in case you have not done so yet.

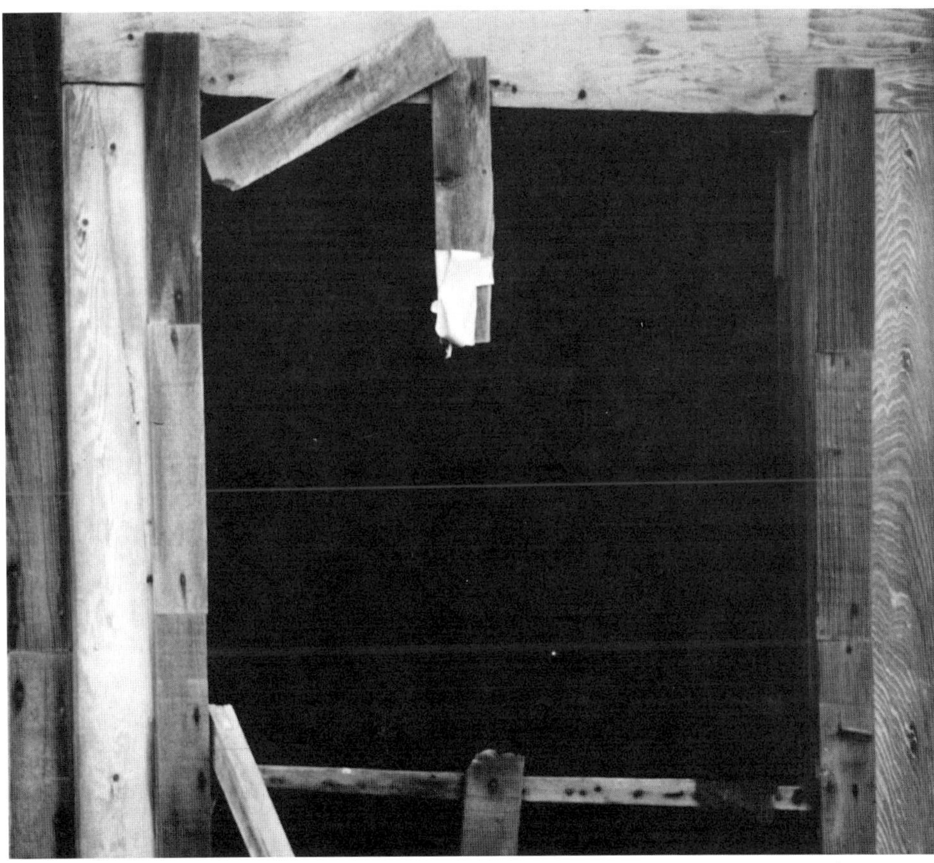

Photo by Thea. Broken barn window—one of my favorites.

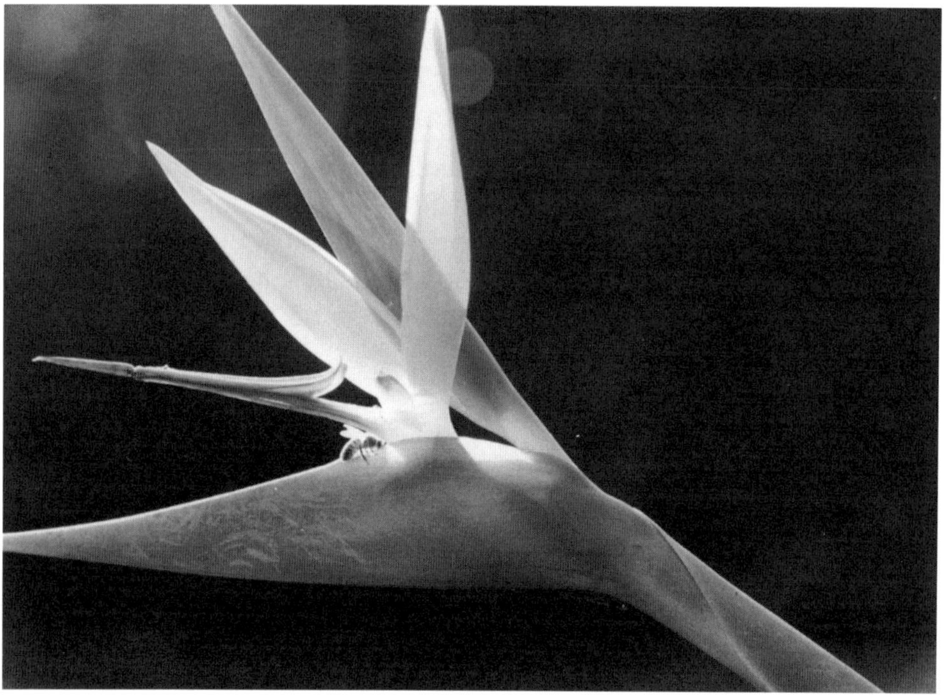

Photo by Thea.

Appendix A

- Chronic Fatigue and The Candida Connection
  By Henry Hoegerman, M.D.
- Homeopathy: A Natural Medicine
  By Dr. Nephtali Solis
- Mercury-Amalgam Toxicity
  By Roy B. Kupsinel, M.D.
- The Double-Blind Test, A Pseudo-Scientific Tool
  By Professor Wolfram Kühnau, M.D.
- The Importance Of Nutrition
  By Steve Boehm, President of Efficient Systems
- Aromatherapy
  By Lucy Campa, Aroma and Massage Therapist
- Live-Cell/Xenotransplant Therapy and CFIDS
  By Professor Wolfram Kühnau, M.D.
- Osteopathy
  By Arlen L. Bass, D.O.
- This I Know
  By Bari Maddock, D.MSc.
- The Possible Connection of Prions and CFIDS
  By Professor Wolfram Kühnau, M.D.

Chronic Fatigue and The Candida Connection

BY HENRY HOEGERMAN, M.D.

In the truest sense, Chronic Fatigue has many contributing factors. One of these factors of no little concern is Candidaisis or, as it is more aptly labeled, "Candida Related Complex."

Candida Related Complex refers to the multiple symptoms related to a chronic (usually unsuspected) gastro-intestinal overgrowth of Candida Albicans and/or related yeast organisms. Let us look first at some of the ways an infection of Candida can produce symptoms, contribute allergic reactions, increase the toxic load the body must deal with, exhaust the biologic defense mechanisms, and impair the immune system.

Anyone who has ever made bread has watched a small amount of yeast placed in a little warm water with sugar added. In a matter of minutes, the yeast comes alive, begins to grow, multiply, and ferment the sugar. The once calm mixture of warm water and sugar becomes active, foaming and bubbling as gas is produced. Picture this happening in the gastro-intestinal tract of a person with an abundance of Candida organisms. It is the very same action: fermentation, gas, and chemical byproducts.

Two of the byproducts so produced are alcohol and chloral hydrate. We all know the effects of alcohol and how it makes us feel, but few are familiar with chloral hydrate. Chloral hydrate is a first-class sedative, well known by doctors. It was also known to the captains of sailing vessels during the clipper ship era of the California gold rush.

Once in California, crew members jumped ship to head for the gold fields. The short-handed captains had a solution to this problem. They bought the sailors a drink at the local bars and laced them with a mixture of morphine and chloral hydrate! The sailors would pass out, only to awaken aboard a ship headed for Shanghai. Thus the expression "the war Shanghaied," and the drink came to be called a "Mickey Finn."

You can readily see how a constant supply of alcohol and chloral hydrate can befuddle the mind, weaken the memory, tax the body's detoxification systems, and directly increase fatigue.

But there is more. The presence of an overgrowth of Candida and yeast in the intestinal tract displaces the normal "good" bacterial flora that is essential to proper digestion. It also has a direct and damaging effect on the cells that line our digestive tract. These cells are responsible for seeing what gets into our body and what is rejected. Just when our digestive system is stressed by the Candida overgrowth displacing our "good" bacteria, our first line of defense is impaired. So it is that protein molecules that are incompletely digested leak through and between the damaged cells that line our intestinal tract.

The immune system "sees" these foreign, incompletely digested proteins and reacts against them. The result becomes food allergies, where none existed before. Toxins that have been digested, as well as Candida itself, likewise find access into our body by the same route.

Another factor causing allergic reactions is the actual presence of Candida. Often, the host will develop an allergy to the Candida and thus become allergic to something they cannot avoid. This, in turn, often involves a crossover allergy to molds and fungi present in the environment, which aggravates the symptoms all the more.

Thus, you see multiple factors by which Candida can add to the burden of the body's detoxification and defense mechanisms and contribute to the final collapse, referred to as Chronic Fatigue and Immune Dysfunction.

How do you determine if a Candida infection is present? It's really quite easy. There are three ways that I know of. The first is to essay the blood for antigens to Candida. If the antigens are high, Candida is suspect. A second is a stool analysis. If Candida organisms can be observed under the microscope, you know they are there. At the same time, you can estimate the amount and the severity of an infection. Also, the stool can be cultured, and often, the Candida will grow out. Then it can be tested to see which medications are effective in killing it, and which are not.

Frankly, I prefer the stool analysis to the blood test. I like to use the actual culture and sensitivity test as a guide to the best treatment. It is surprising how different strains of Candida show resistance to different medications. One word of caution about the stool analysis: most local labs do not do a good job of finding Candida, so work with a doctor familiar with treating Candida and the specialty laboratories that do stool analysis. Personally, I use Great Smokies Diagnostic Laboratory. They specialize in stool analysis, and I find the results very satisfactory.

The third way to test for Candida is the "clinical test." Basically, this means that you suspect Candida and treat the patient accordingly. If the symptoms improve, then the diagnosis is confirmed. The advantage of this method is that it saves time and money, plus if it works, you've solved the problem. The disadvantage is that if you choose a treatment to which the Candida virus is resistant, Candida may be ruled out, when in reality the Candida is present, but the therapy is ineffective.

Candidaisis is not a simple problem that can be solved by giving the patient a drug and killing a "bug" and that's it. It will always be there, the question is do you have it under control? So the treatment involves reducing the number of Candida organisms, and then keeping the number (and thus their effect) at a minimum for a period of time. During this time, it is essential to maximize the patient's immune system and total body health. Then, hopefully, their defenses will be successful in keeping the Candida under control.

Although this sounds simple in such few words, the case is not so. All the factors that weaken and overburden the detoxification and defense system of the body must be addressed and removed. At the same time, the general health, strength, and vitality of each cell in the body must be nourished (and nourished is the correct word) for maximal strength, health, and performance.

With these thoughts in mind, I would advise the Candida patient to work with a well-rounded physician familiar with the Candida problem and the alternative medical field, as well. In my experience, I have seen too many patients looking for the magic cure, trying everything they can. Proper therapy involves a more comprehensive approach. This is especially true when Candida is associated with Chronic Fatigue and Immune Dysfunction.

A quick list of some of the areas where treatment may be directed would include the following: mental and emotional stress; the body burden of toxic chemicals and heavy metals (e.g. amalgam dental fillings containing mercury); vitamin, mineral, enzyme, amino acid, or essential fatty acid deficiency; thyroid function; chronic adrenal insufficiency; depressed immune function; intestinal parasites and bacteria; malabsorption and "leaky gut" syndrome; or chronic liver detoxification overload. It takes an involved patient working together with a knowledgeable professional to put it all together.

There are some specific ways to directly approach the Candida problem. First is the diet. There are several "Candida diets" outlined in books available on the subject. Most are a little difficult to follow. To make things simple, and in my mind the most important single item is to AVOID SUGAR. Remember how yeast ferments when placed in warm sugar water?

Every Candida patient should avoid sugar. Besides nourishing Candida, and causing it to rapidly multiply, sugar in its own right has an adverse effect on the immune system. So read the diets in the books dealing with the subject if you wish, but always AVOID SUGAR.

The next step in treatment is the use of drugs to kill the Candida organisms. The old standby is Nystatin. Nystatin has been around for years and years and has a good track record. Nystatin is a very safe drug, in that it is not absorbed into the body. It does its work in the intestinal tract; thus, it rarely produces any side effects and can be used for a long period of time. However, Candida can invade the wall of the intestinal tract and hide here from Nystatin. Also, if there is systemic involvement, Nystatin will not reach it.

Three potent drugs work very well. They are Nizerol (ketocomazole), Diflucan (fluconazole), and Sporanox (itraconazole). They are all absorbed by the body and attack Candida wherever it may lurk. They are usually strong, fast, and effective. There are drawbacks, however. They all can have a toxic effect on the liver, and death has been reported with the use of Nizerol. So their usage needs to be monitored closely with liver function tests. Diflucan and Sporanox are on the expensive side, which sometimes limits their use. Nevertheless, they are very useful drugs. However, I have seen cases where the strain of Candida was resistant to all three.

In addition to drugs, there are some very useful herbs. Among these is our old friend garlic, which has been known to be lethal to Candida. Others include grapefruit seed extract, Caprylic Acid, Undecylenic Acid, Berberine, Tannalbit, and Uva-ursi. Although these can usually be obtained over the counter, I would not advise self-medication. In fact, in any event, I like to see a culture of the stool tested for effectiveness of various antifungal agents to allow the selection of the most useful and least toxic agent.

The next thing to think about, after killing the Candida, is to replenish the normal flora, the "good" bacteria, that belong in the intestinal tract. To do this, ample dosages of lactobacillus, acidophillus, and related enteric bacteria are required. These preparations are available at any health food store. There are many different brands to choose from, most of them very satisfactory, and most claiming to be superior to the rest. It is a reasonable approach to alternate from brand to brand to ensure as wide a variety of replacement bacteria as possible.

At the same time you are killing the Candida bacteria and replacing the normal bacterial flora, a good nutritional program is a must. As mentioned earlier, restoration of the immune system is important, and this requires optimal nutrition for each and every cell in the body. The subject is too extensive to include here. A nutritional program is best based on individual studies such as a hair analysis for minerals, trace elements, and amino acids. This will show which nutrients you may need more or less of. Here, again, you need the help of a professional.

Without doubt, if Candida organisms are present, proper therapy for this problem is a must in the resolution of Chronic Fatigue and Immune Dysfunction.

Homeopathy: A Natural Medicine

By Dr. Nephtali Solis

One of the many treatment modalities available to us under the heading of alternative medicine is homeopathy, a medical science that uses natural substances as healing agents. This medical art is presently being practiced by both professional homeopaths and laypersons all over the world. Homeopathy was once widely used in the United States up to about seventy-five years ago, when it was unfortunately displaced in favor of what is now called modern scientific medicine. However, homeopathy survived, being practiced in a smaller scale, and is now again gaining favor by regular medicine and the public at large.

One of the appealing factors in homeopathy is that the medicine itself does not contain any chemical substances, but is a medicine that is derived from the energies of natural substances, such as plants, minerals, animals, tissues, etc. The purpose of homeopathy is to stimulate the body's own immune resources to strengthen organs and tissues, thereby bringing about an energetic balance within the organism. It is important to remember that these medicines do not produce toxic side effects as conventional drug therapy tends to do.

The action of homeopathy, which was formulated by Dr. Samuel Hahnemann in Germany about 200 years ago, is to detoxify the body from its own homo-toxins, that is, toxic byproducts as a result of physiological processes, to strengthen organ and organ tissues by rejecting pathogens, such as bacteria, viruses, fungi, chemicals, and other noxious agents that are found in our households and environment, and to bring about harmony in the organism through a self-healing mechanism.

It is through this ongoing detoxification of tissues and organs that the body re-establishes its own energetic balance and brings about a former state of "ease," provided that the body's own immune system is sufficiently strong to bring about this change. If homeopathy is prescribed cautiously, choosing the proper remedies, even in a weakened system, healing can take place over a period of time. Not only are homo-toxins burdening the body, but also pathogens, such as viruses, bacteria, fungi, chemicals, etc. Therefore, it is of paramount importance that in any treatment program, in acute or chronic disease, pathogens should also be extricated from the system in addition to all other supportive therapies, otherwise the organs are not allowed to heal.

Dr. Hahnemann's healing principle of "like cures like" is similar to the idea that you "fight fire with fire." The action of homeopathy is based on the principle that if a substance that is introduced into a healthy body causes symptoms of a particular nature, this same substance will cure an individual exhibiting the same type of symptoms that are characteristic of that substance. This has been called the "law of similars" and is the basic principle of homeopathy.

In choosing the proper homeopathy remedy (the more commonly used term for medicine in homeopathy), the practitioner has to assess the entire system as in the case in both Oriental and Ayurvedic medicines. This is the basis of holistic medicine since it is the pathological, mental, emotional, and spiritual aspects of the individual that have to be treated in order to bring about complete healing. It is the treatment of the root of the problem, rather than treating the symptoms alone, that gradually brings about complete healing.

Within homeopathy, there are various approaches to treatment. A "classical" approach would be one in which a single remedy is chosen that will treat the symptom complex of the individual, whether one or several subsequent doses are given. A more "modern" approach would be one in which several remedies are given at one time, in addition to a single remedy that also treats the total symptom complex. It is extremely important to choose a remedy, called the "constitutional," that will also address the emotional imbalance in the individual so that a harmony is again created between the limbic system, the body's emotional center, and the immune system, since it is the latter system that protects it at all times from pathogens invading the deeper tissues of the body.

It is of equal importance that, in addition to the constitutional remedy, nosodes be given. Nosodes are specially prepared homeopathic remedies made from any pathogens such as viruses, bacteria, etc. If the liver and the kidneys, major organs of detoxification, as well as the pancreas, are treated with nosodes, then the cells and supportive tissues of these cells and organs will be burdened beyond repair.

As we know, any system of treatment and healing is a gradual process, and homeopathy is no exception. However, under ideal circumstances, where the individual is willing to accept healing and the proper remedies are given in addition to other supportive therapies, the healing results can be amazing at the end of the treatment program.

One of my very dear patients whom I have treated over the past several years is Thea Schlosser. It has been an honor and a source of gratification to be able to be part of her healing medical team. Looking back, I have been able to see her progress, knowing that she will be able to return to her creative life and work that she loves in the near future. She is truly a "patient patient," who has a righteous and altruistic spirit and who has been a source of inspiration to many. I am indeed grateful to her and honored by her allowing me to contribute this small article to her timely, resourceful, and inspirational book.

Dr. Solis is a homeopath, an acupuncturist, and a physical therapist who has practiced in Santa Barbara for the past thirty years. He was instrumental in establishing the first homeopathic store in Santa Barbara.
He can be reached at (805) 682-7103 or faxed at (805) 687-7936. An (800) number will soon be available.

Mercury-Amalgam Toxicity

By Roy B. Kupsinel, M.D.

From the London MAIL on November 13, 1983: "Wife Gets Her Sight Back at Dentist's: Sweden..." Blind housewife Gun Toresoon regained her vision at age 43 after being blind since the age of 20. She had her dentist remove three heavily filled teeth! In 1981, a pre-dental student, David Harden, 21, developed rheumatoid arthritis. The prescribed drug therapy gradually became ineffective. His father, a dentist too, removed two amalgam fillings from one tooth and that was the end of David's rheumatoid arthritis. Roy B. Kupsinel, M.D., suffered from severe headaches since the placing of his first fillings of mercury-amalgam when he was about five years old. At age sixty-three, he has been almost headache-free for nine years. He had twenty-nine fillings removed and replaced with composites, ceramic plastic resin material!

THE AMALGAM WARS

The dental silver-mercury amalgam has been in existence for 165 years! The first of the three amalgam wars broke out in the United States in the 1840s. The American Society of Dental Surgeons required its members to sign an agreement not to put amalgam in a patient's mouth. Members violated their agreement, the organization dissolved, and the American Dental Association was born. Yes, more than 150 years ago, some wise individuals realized the dangers of the toxicity of amalgams, which contain approximately 50% mercury initially! The second amalgam war was fought in Europe and especially Germany! A German chemist, Dr. Alfred Stock, introduced the concept of "micromercurialism," mercury affecting the individual cells on a physiological level. Having suffered from severe mercury toxicity, Stock published a startling article in 1926 in a scientific journal. Recently, it was translated by Mats Hanson into English and published in the Journal of Orthmolecular Psychiatry. Why are so many dentists today unfamiliar with Stock's work? Is it being taught in our dental schools? The third amalgam war is being waged now with its inception in the 1970s. It is on a professional, scientific, and public level with consumer movements in Sweden, West Germany, and the United States.

THE ESCAPE OF MERCURY FROM AMALGAMS

In 1957, Frykholm concluded that when saliva covers the amalgam, the mercury is no longer released. His conclusion has been disproved. Yet the minds of many establishment dentists remain shrouded in ignorance.

Scientists have shown as much as fifteen-fold increase in the mercury vapor after chewing. The Jerome Mercury Vapor Analyzer is an instrument that is gaining acceptance by many dentists. It is specific for mercury and vividly impresses the patient with the dramatic increase in the mercury vapor after chewing sugarless gum for ten to fifteen minutes.

Old amalgams still contain about 28% or slightly greater that half of their original 50% mercury. They are like a time-release capsule, releasing vapors, particles, and ions twenty-four hours a day—often for several years!

MERCURY EXCRETION

The routes of elimination of mercury are the urine, stool, lungs, bile, sweat, and saliva. Sauna baths include sweating and are beneficial. Kidney function is disturbed within minutes after mercury enters the blood stream. Its first effect is increased urination and, if extensive damage occurs, urinary output may decrease and even stop because of kidney failure. It is incorrect to equate the excretion of the mercury in the urine to that given off by amalgam.

STANDARD FOR SAFE LEVELS?

In a nutshell, mercury is highly toxic to humans and, therefore, any amount is harmful to the cells and tissues of human beings. Mercury can occur in elemental, inorganic, and organic forms. "Safe" levels of exposure have titles such as Threshold Limit Values (THV) and Maximum Allowable Concentrations (MAC).

Since mercury enters the body from the fillings via the lungs and the intestinal tract and travels via the circulatory system all over the human organism, it is possible to have just about any other symptom from this poison. Here are a few more examples: loss of self-confidence, shyness, shortened attention span, fits of anger, insomnia, drowsiness, abdominal cramps, diarrhea, colitis, persistent cough, emphysema, shallow breathing, muscle weakness, fatigue, anemia, swelling or edema, loss of appetite, loss of weight, and obesity that does not respond well to weight reduction programs.

DIAGNOSIS AND TREATMENT

If the doctor and patients are in agreement without testing that mercury is toxic to the patient's body, then there is no need for testing with one exception. Some authorities feel that the electro-galvanic test or current potential in order to determine the sequence for amalgam removal is quite helpful and important in order to avoid a flare-up of neurological problems.

The removal of dental mercury is not a "cure," rather it is the removal from the body of a very toxic substance. If the physical symptoms of an unknown cause are alleviated by the removal, all the better. Amalgam removal does not remove mercury that is already compelled in the body. Yet once the last amalgam is removed, the body will begin to eliminate the complexed mercury, and increased urinary mercury levels are frequently seen. Detoxification therapy may be necessary before relief of symptoms is accomplished. I compare the mercury-amalgam problem with the source from the fillings and the accumulation in the body organs and tissues to a bathtub with a running faucet, and a closed drain. By removing the amalgams, turning off the faucet the source of the mercury is eliminated. By pulling the plug, cheating or clawing out the mercury by nutritional supplementation, the body is drained of the mercury contamination!

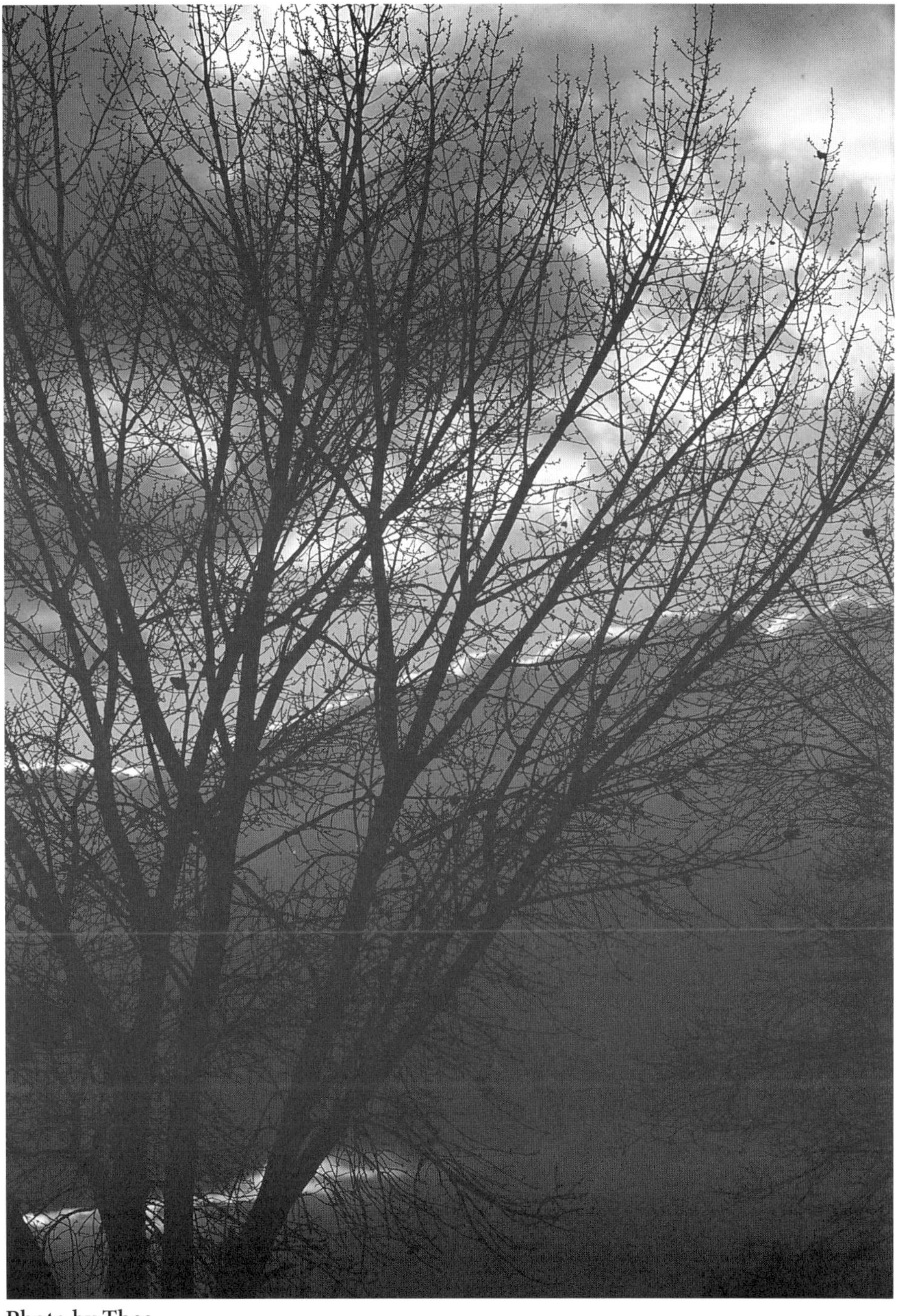

Photo by Thea.

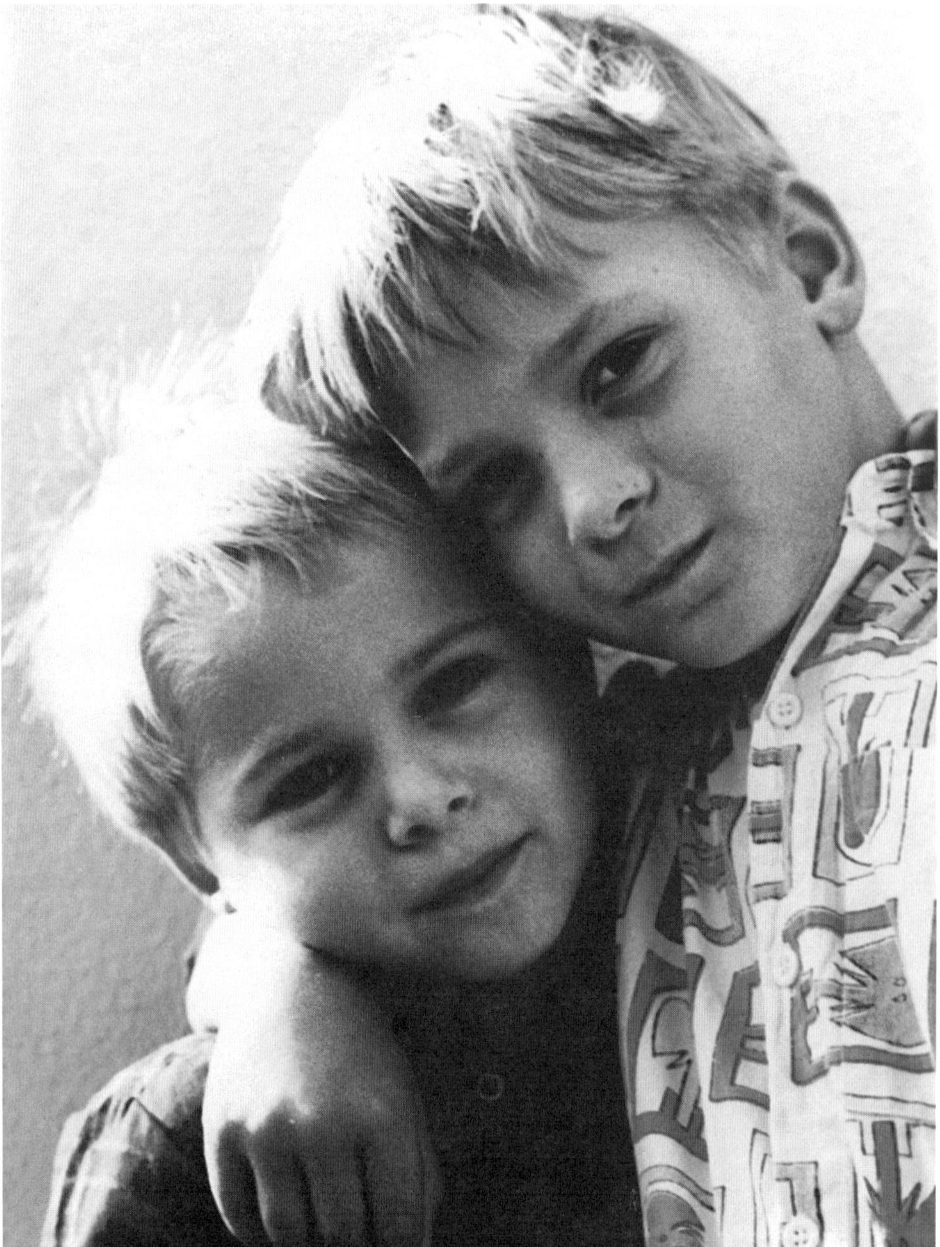

My dear grandsons Ryan and Jeff Boehm, Ingrid and Steve's two sons. We are unique—all of us. These are two of my angels. Jeff has asthma, Ryan does not. Why? Dr. Kühnau makes a very valuable point with his article, The Double-Blind Test.

APPENDIX A

The Double-Blind Test, A Pseudo-Scientific Tool

BY PROFESSOR WOLFRAM KÜHNAU, M.D.

It is remarkable that a certain philosophy can mislead humanity over centuries, as is the case in the statements of the famous French philosopher Descartes (Cartesius) three centuries ago. He insisted that we can separate the body and soul as early as in the Aristotelian and early Medieval Christian philosophy, and late Medieval church leaders (Thomas Aquinas and others) postulated this again and again.

Now, astonishingly enough, in our "modern" time, this basic error is still continuing to work and is regarded as a fundamental truth. One of the misleading examples to try to petrify by being "scientific" is the so-called "double-blind test." Any new pharmaceutical product to be admitted to the market has to undergo this proof.

Every doctor knows how very important is the belief of the patient that the medicine the doctor prescribed will help him, and the personality of the doctor plays an important role in the success of the treatment. That is a fact. But instead of accepting this fact the still Medieval, orthodox medicine has found a new way of "scientific authentic exact determination" of the borders between body and soul.

The enchanting key word is "placebo." This Latin word means, "I will do a favor to the patient." So this substitute has to look and smell quite the same way as the original product; the only difference is that it has to not have any efficiency at all. Now, the patient has to believe that he is taking the original product, and, indeed, this "zero" sometimes has some remarkable success.

If I take two groups of patients, one will get the true product and the other the placebo. The subtraction of the "placebo effect" from the results is then considered the "real efficiency." For example, if the placebo had an efficiency of 30% and the true product 70%, the definitive effect is 40%. It seems very understandable and scientific, especially since the doctor distributing both products does not himself know which is which. Seems to be very correct. Is it true?

These "scientific people" are offering one more thing. To equalize some possible differences in the individual situations of the patient, the scientists take a large number of patients, for example two hundred (two groups of one hundred each), so that they are randomized. This gives us the "randomized double-blind test."

Now, let us take asthma as an example. Asthma can have different causes, including problems in the back bones of the chest, chronic tonsillitis, wrong composition of the intestinal microbes, or even psychological stress. Is it possible to randomize these things? If one group has fifty women of over 50, the other group must be the same. Is it possible that they all have the same type of asthma? I don't think so!

Then, it is the law that the doctor has to ask the patient if they are willing to participate in the double-blind test, so the patient is prepared that perhaps he is getting the placebo. Of course, the doctor giving the "medicine" does not know which is the true medicine and which is the placebo, but he is also biased in a certain sense.

In addition, if the doctor is a young, caring optimistic man, the effect of the same drug, or placebo will not be the same as if the doctor is not a very kind person. The same test, with the same patients but different doctors, will have different results, depending on the personality of the doctor. Is this a scientific test? It is not! Neglecting the fact that we cannot separate the body from the soul, that they are an inseparable entity, these tests cover ignorance with arrogance! This cannot be allowed.

Also, the double-blind test is immoral! An example is the publication on the so-called inefficiency of the application of Laetrile. One hundred patients with terminal cancer were given Laetrile, while the other hundred were given nothing (a placebo). This leaves one hundred patients untreated, possibly to die, only to prove a scientific question. This is not only immoral, it is a crime.

So, the double-blind test is not only useless, it is against any medical responsibility. The German Professor Martini pointed out in the '30s that one very well documented case can be more instructive than one hundred statistics. We have enough serious medical tests that allow definite conclusions. We humans are not rabbits. We don't need the pseudo-scientific double-blind test!

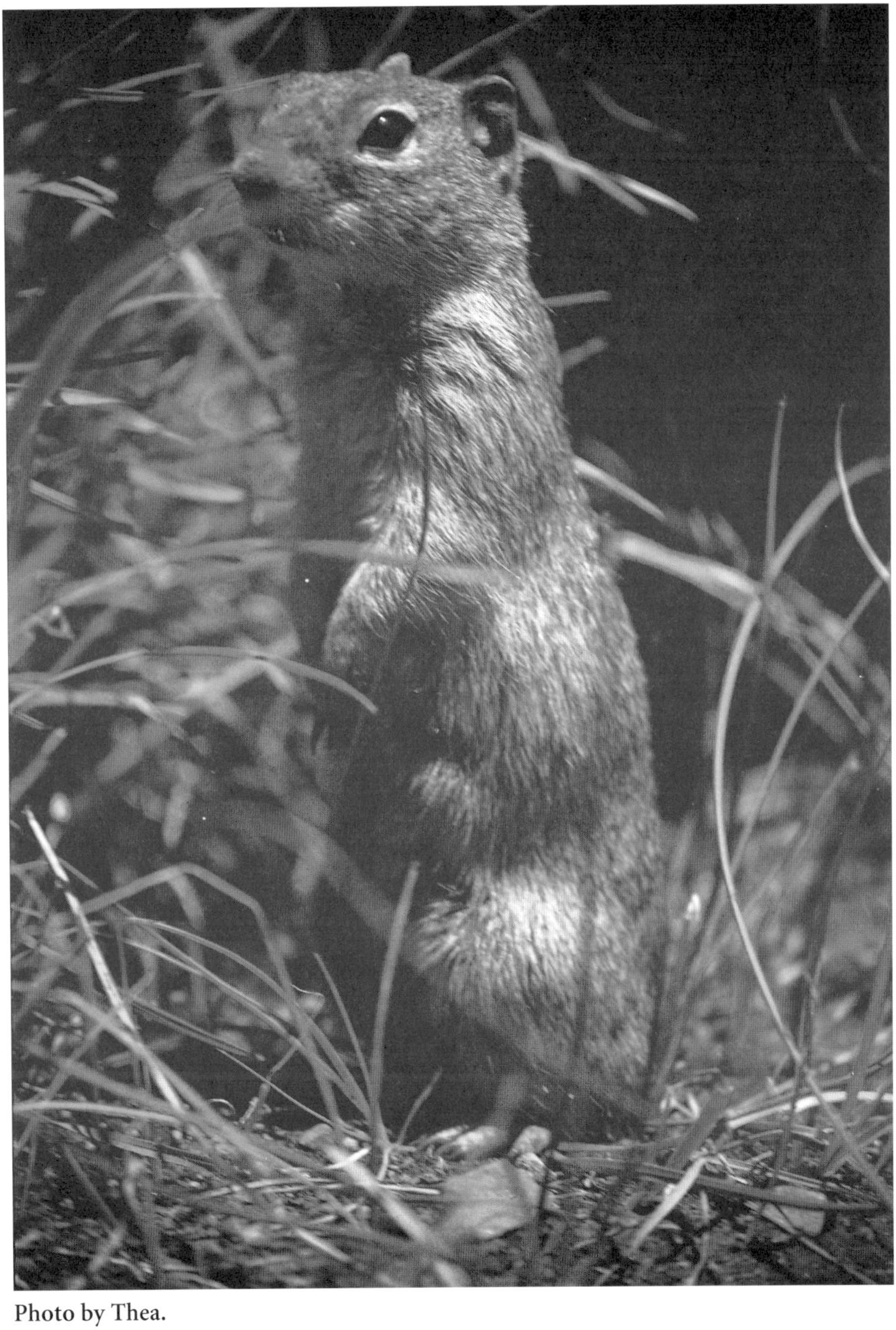

Photo by Thea.

The Importance Of Nutrition

By Steve Boehm, President of Efficient Systems
665 Coyote Road, Santa Barbara, CA 93108
(805) 969-4948

Toward the end of 1993, my mother-in-law Thea Schlosser convinced me that I should try the multi-vitamins she was taking. I thought I was getting everything I needed from the foods I was eating. I learned an important lesson: there are many levels of health, ranging from poor to optimal. When I found myself feeling better than ever taking the multi-vitamins, I decided to investigate and determine the best nutritional supplements and health products for my own family's use.

Even a well-balanced, nutritious diet does not give us the vitamins, minerals, and other important nutrition it once did. The commercialization of agriculture yields larger crops, while sacrificing nutritional value. This is compounded by our current environment with chemicals, pollution, radiation, and stress. The answer is not to turn to synchronized vitamins, but to take superfoods and concentrated foods. Researchers at the National Cancer Institute and other scientists have launched million-dollar campaigns to identify foods that enhance our immune systems. They are scouring the globe for foods and plants with anti-cancer compounds. In the cover story "Better than Vitamins" found in *Newsweek,* it is asserted that, "It is whole foods...that pack the disease-preventing wallop. That's because they harbor a whole ratatouille of compounds that have never seen the inside of a vitamin bottle...the compounds are called phytochemicals....In the world where science merges with health, phytochemicals are the next big thing."

With so many product choices, where should you begin?

Thea asked me to offer the following products. She did this because she knows first-hand of my commitment to helping people, the considerable research I have undertaken, and because she has personally been using these products successfully for the past year. The steps are:

1) Build an energy foundation with superfoods:
   Micro and Marine Algae Blend [1]

10002 Full Spectrum Algae	120 tabs	(15-day supply)	$17.00
10003 Full Spectrum Algae	240 tabs	(30-day supply)	$27.00

2) Follow the Three Golden Keys to Health:
   First, add internal protection from potentially infectious organisms. Protection from illness and disease starts from within. Beneficial flora in your intestinal tract wards off disease-causing bacteria.

10031 Inner Youth	60 tabs	(30-60 days)	$26.00
10032 Inner Youth	120 tabs	(60-90 days)	$38.00

   Second, improve energy and digestion with enzymes to get more from the food you eat.

10041 FooZymes	90 capsules	(30+ days)	$20.00

   Third, boost antioxidant protection against lifestyle stress and cellular damage.

10050 Healthy Cells	180 tablets	(30 days)	$25.00
60001 JuicePlus [2]	120 tablets	(30 days)	$46.00

All products are backed by a money-back guarantee. All orders will receive information about the other unique and beneficial products we carry.

Thank you, Steve, for your invaluable information and your efforts to help others.
I would like to share my experience with the exercise machine offered by Efficient Systems. You simply lie down on the floor, place you legs over the exerciser, and turn it on. It gently rocks your entire body up to fifteen minutes, which is roughly equivalent to a 1.5-mile walk. For $480.00, I feel it is one of the best investments I've made for my well-being. I personally wouldn't want to be without it and would recommend this machine to anybody who is not able to exercise regularly due to an illness, such as CFIDS. It is simple and effective. After I use this machine, I feel more alert, and my general pain is decreased.

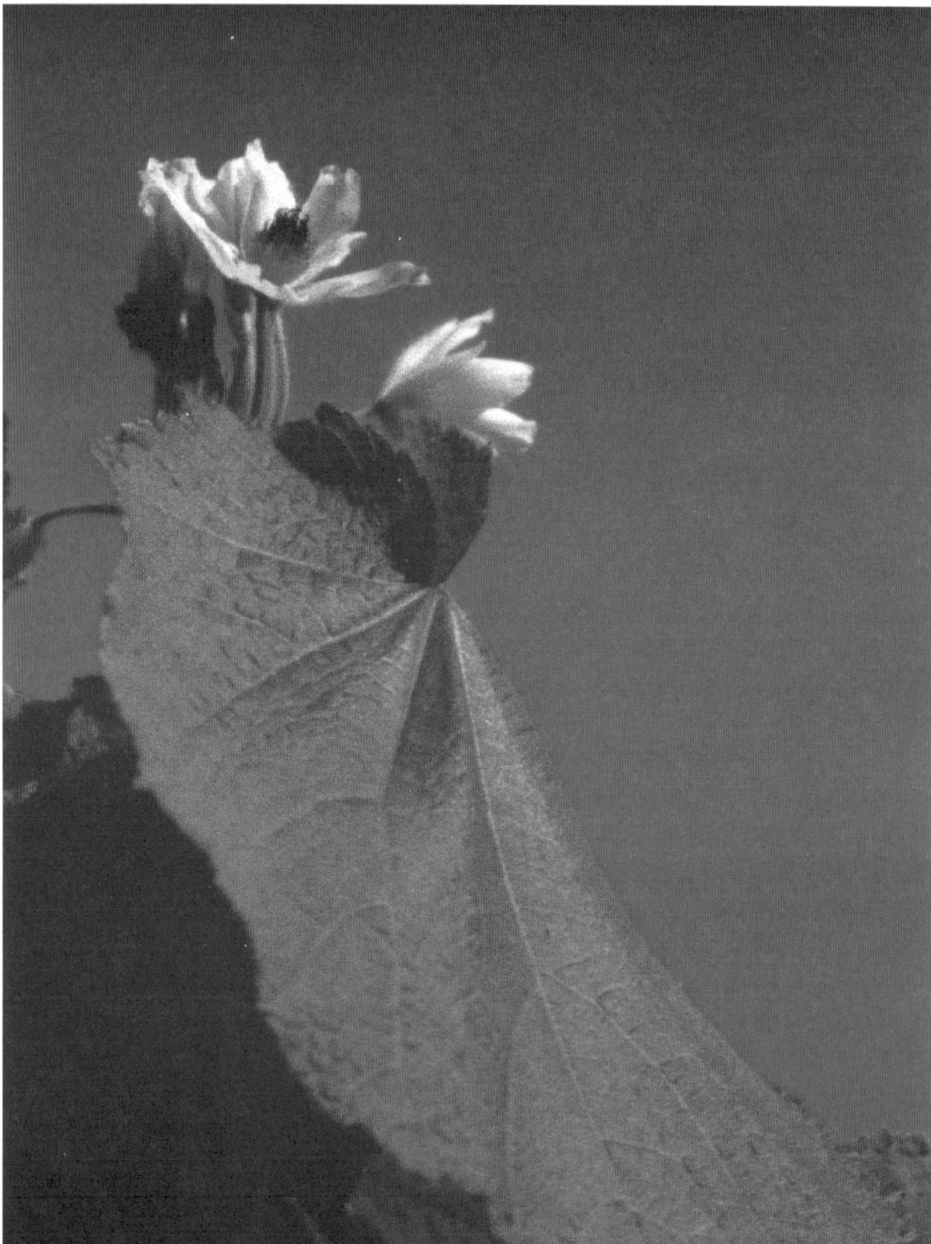

Photo by Thea.

Aromatherapy

By Lucy Campa, Aroma and Massage Therapist

Essential oils are vibrational. When massaged onto the body, they penetrate the skin. The small molecular structure allows this. An essential oil massage should be done with an intention. As I start treatment, my energies along with the oils chosen to heal the imbalance work together. Prayer also plays a big part in the effectiveness of the treatment, and somehow a shift takes place within my client. The more the client relaxes and allows the energy of the oils to penetrate, the more effectively they work.

Essential oils are wonderful for stress-related problems and, if used continuously, will help in curing countless problems, including PMS, muscle strain, insomnia, and digestive disorders. Aromatherapy also relieves the emotions of anger, fear, and the "I just feel like I am going crazy" syndrome so often encountered because of our hectic lifestyles.

Essential oils are very effective in the bath, applied during massage, or diffused into the air. Both children and adults respond well to treatment with essential oils and seem to avoid illnesses if treated early.

Essential oils are great mood enhancers and are the guiding light needed when you want to slip into a quiet meditation.

The list of benefits encountered goes on. How could anyone go wrong using natural plant extracts as a way of healing? I call it getting back to smelling the flowers and taking responsibility for one's health.

Lucy is my Aroma and Massage Therapist. I was very surprised about aromatherapy's healing abilities. I have also found it convenient to order oils from Lucy and treat myself according to how I feel. If you are interested in learning more about aromatherapy, Lucy can be reached at:
523 Brinkerhoff Ave., Santa Barbara, CA 93101, (805) 564-8465

Live-Cell/Xenotransplant Therapy and CFIDS

By Professor Wolfram Kühnau, M.D.

The hippocampus, located in the limbic system and close to the hypothalamus, is known as the place where memory is entered with calcium and NDM asparatase and also the place where interleukin 2 is produced, which then stimulates the production of killer cells in the bone marrow and is also involved in Chronic Fatigue Syndrome (CFS).

When the production of Interleukin 2 in the hippocampus is higher than normal and in the bone marrow the production of killer cells is paradoxically drastically depressed, there will be an interruption of the communication between the hippocampus and the bone marrow in the system of messenger-receptor. The question must then be asked as to the cause of this interruption.

Both myself and Katzentstein have suggested that an early childhood brain trauma could be responsible. But it is entirely possible that there could be other causes. I hypothesize that an irritation of the sympathetic network of the neck, for example, resulting from whiplash, could lead to overactivity of the pineal gland and the subsequent suppression of the communication between the hippocampus and the bone marrow.

A systematic investigation of CFS patients indicates that a high percentage of them have a history of neck and vertebrae injury. This would appear to indicate that not only the hyper-function of the pineal gland can be important, but also a hyper-function can cause severe disturbances. Osteopathic or chiropractic treatment has been shown to help CFS patients.

Let us now review the practical conclusions we have reached regarding live cell therapy.

1) It is imperative for the doctor to be assured that live cells are practically free of any risk when given in reasonable and consistent quantities. The horror stories about complications voiced by the enemies of this modality have resulted from unbelievable overdoses and carelessness of application by unqualified people seeking large profits with this revolutionary therapy. The German government and

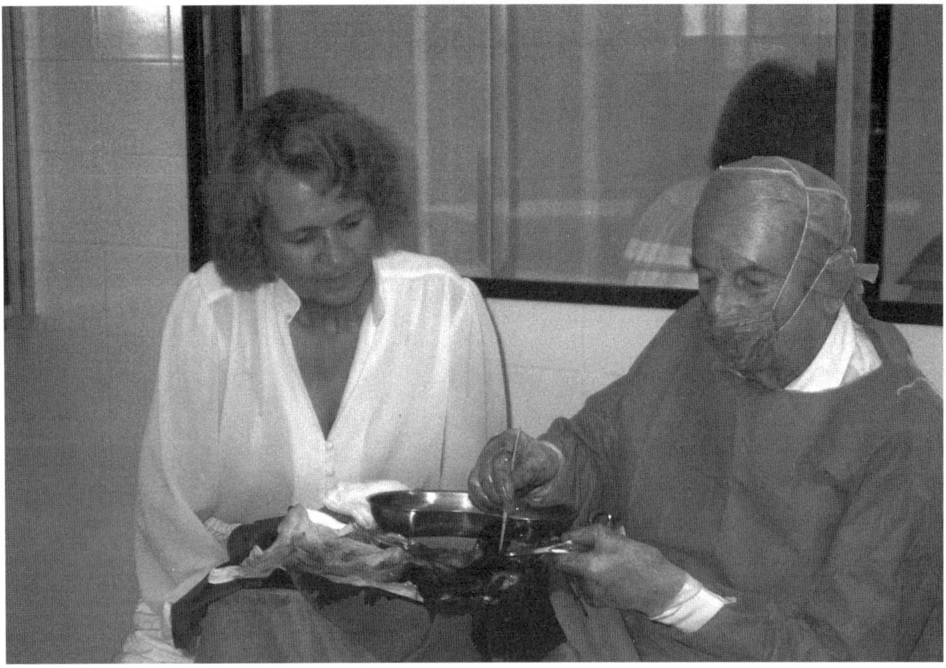

In 1994, I conducted an interview with Professor Dr. Wolfram Kühnau as he prepared cells from a shark embryo that were later to be used in xenotransplant therapy. Professor Kühnau only uses embryos from pregnant sharks caught by fishermen.

other concerned countries were absolutely correct in stopping these unconscionable procedures. It cannot be stressed too strongly that the therapy must be administered only by very experienced and conscientious doctors. This is cardinal rule number one.

2) There must never be more than six different cells given in one treatment. Booster shots must not be given before six months have elapsed. Naturally, there can be exceptions to this, but only in a minimum of cases and on an individual basis. The only true exception is in the treatment of cancer.

3) If a prospective patient is suffering an infection, i.e., sinusitis, etc., treatment must be postponed until the infection is cleared.

4) The patient must rest for at least two days after the treatment. During this time he must avoid the sun, hot baths or showers, and any type of enzymes (for example, papayas). After two days, the patient should take on a daily basis 10 grams (10,000 mg) of vitamin

C for a period of three weeks. After the three-week regimen, he can reduce the vitamin C intake to a lower dosage. Vitamin C is useful in building up new synapses (connections) from nerve fibers.

5) The effect of the live-cell therapy is usually not apparent for four to six weeks after treatment. In some cases, the effect can be even after. On the other hand, some patients will experience beneficial effects much earlier. Each individual responds differently.

6) There is not "the asthma," the "psoriasis," "the stomach," etc., so there is not, as has been recommended by some doctors, a particular combination of cells for a particular disease. We urgently warn against these false prophets. Every patient has his own history, and we always must seek the cause, not the symptom. A number of different causes can lead to the same disease. If we treat the cause, the disease will disappear in a high percentage of cases. If it does not (which is rare), find out why.

There can be, as Dr. Hunecke ponted out, a "disturbance field" such as, for example, an old scar or a chronic misdiagnosed sinus infection or a disorder in the neck vertebrae; therefore live cell treatment demands the highest quality medical knowledge and responsibility. But it is the first time that we can regulate a hormonal disorder. By using hormones, we are treating only a symptom and by suppressing the immune system, we subject the patient to a lifetime of drug usage. Not so with live-cell therapy.

Together with Professor Staudinger, I proved clearly in twenty-four urinalysis tests that through the use of live-cell therapy, a low hormone level rose to normal limits and a too-high hormone level decreased to normal levels. This is what I like to call "harmonization." It can be likened to a conductor and his orchestra. Prior to live cell therapy, this was not possible.

Now we can scientifically prove beyond any doubt that the embryonic cellular material is brought through our macrophages (respectively the main organelles such as the ribosomes, lysosomes, microsomes, mitochondria, etc.) to the human target organ. We know, too, that this material will be accepted by the body as its own and not be rejected as being foreign. Further, if the application is made reasonably and properly, there are never any severe side effects.

For the first time, we now have an idea of how this happens. It

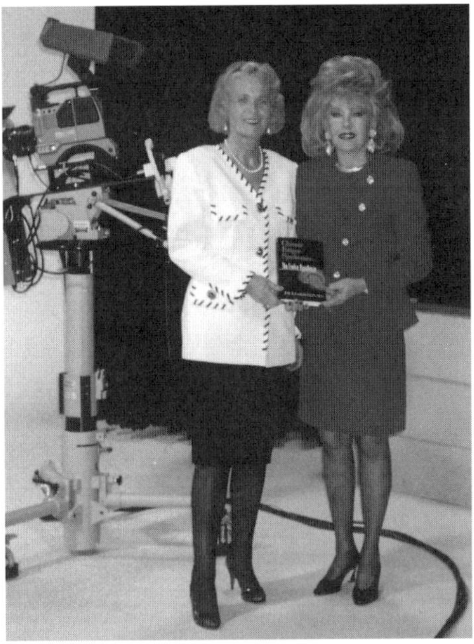

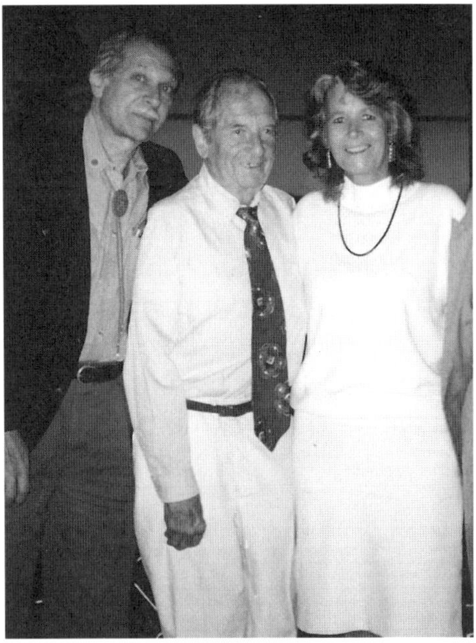

Left: (from left) Thea Schlosser and Mrs. Elisa Henley Frerra, TV producer and host, "Growing Younger," after a TV interview regarding CFIDS with Jay Goldstein, M.D. Right: (from left) Roy Kupsinel, M.D., Prof. W. Kühnau, M.D., and Thea Schlosser. Dr. Kupsinel is former owner of *Health Conscious* Magazine.

involves the so-called "factors." The most famous of these is the nerve growth factor, discovered by the Nobel prize-winner Dr. Rita Levi Montalcini of Rome. Then there is the hepatopoetic factor (Dr. Ruhenstroth, Frankfurt); then the skin growth factor and now the fibroblast growth factor. We can compare these factors to zip codes in our mailing system.

The most fascinating and surprising aspect of all this, and one that was never suspected, is that these factors are almost identical in all of nature. In other words, in the frog and in the human, they are the same. With this new knowledge, I hypothesize that in the future we can prepare for a heart transplant by an injection of animal heart cells a certain time before, and by so doing, we can hopefully educate the immune system of the patient to tolerate and accept the actual transplant rather than attempting to reject it. If this proves true, the immune suppressers—as, for example, cyclostorine or the better tolerated FK 506 (Dr. Starlz, Pittsburg)—will no longer be necessary.

So—the heart of a baboon to save a human's life? So far, so good. I have no intention of entering into a discussion of the moral consequences.

Rather, we are here discussing the biological and medical consequences of new biological and biochemical knowledge. A serious consideration should be that a patient living with the baboon heart would be dependent on immune-suppressing drugs for an entire lifetime. Further, this patient will live in a situation very comparable to having AIDS. For his entire lifetime, this patient is susceptible to such infections as pneumocystosis.

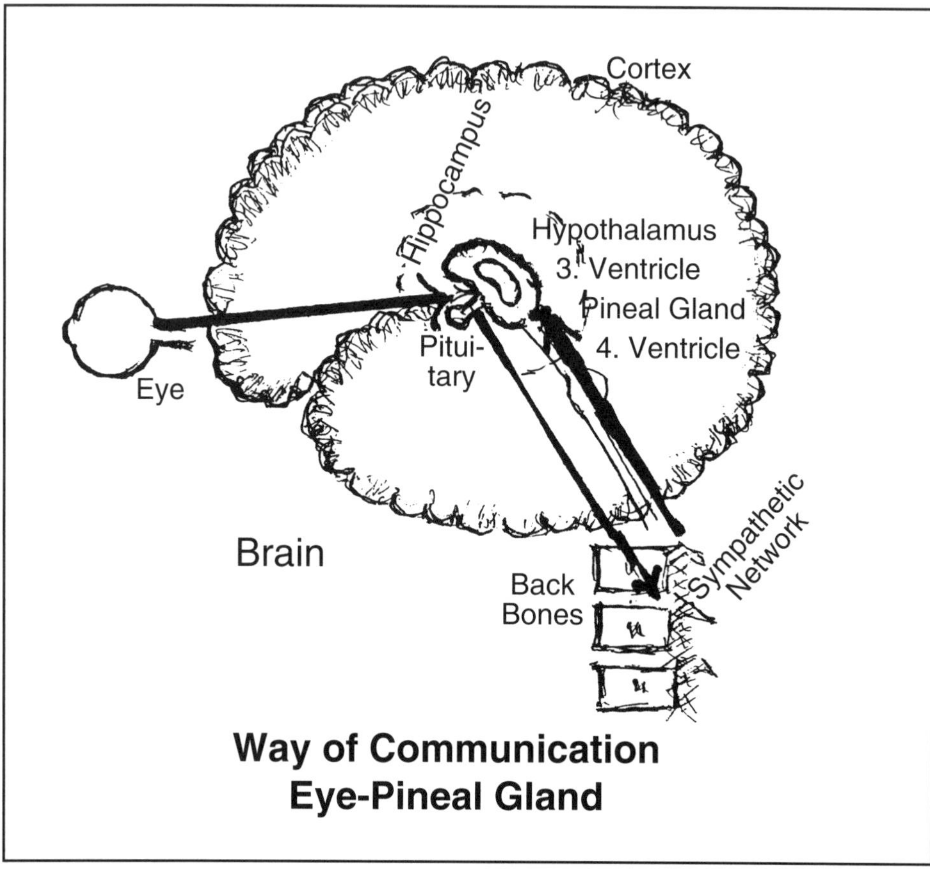

A sketch of the brain showing the pineal gland by Professor Dr. W. Kühnau.

Let us consider those animals having comparable pregnancy or gestation times with humans. During the first three months of pregnancy, these embryos will not develop any immune activity. So, again, this embryonic material will be tolerated by humans very readily. There will be no rejection by the human host.

Let us further consider an incredible possibility. Suppose there are animals in which the fetus, during the first three months, has organs of the same size as a human adult. Those three-month fetal animal organs would be well tolerated as transplants into humans. Let us imagine a heart from a whale fetus during the third month of pregnancy. This is approximately the same size as a human heart and would be tolerated very well as a transplant by humans. The recipient would have no side effects and would not need any immune suppressers. This is truly futuristic thinking.

Or consider a preparatory animal-embryonic-tissue-transplant before the transplant of the human heart of a donator with an embryonic heart of approximately the same size as the human heart. With this excursion into a future dreamworld, we now come back to reality.

Live-cell therapy will only be effective if corresponding tissue in the human body is still available. It may be weakened, but it must still be living so that it can respond to a tissue transplant of the same organ. This is why the famous experiment of Dr. Madrazo Navarro in Mexico did not have a lasting effect. The brain has no adrenal cells that could respond. Let us review. Dr. Navarro transplanted adrenal tissue into the brain of Parkinson's patients with an initial good result. However, it was a short-lived success, because the transplant worked only so long as the transplanted cells were alive. Thus it is clear: the consequence is that implants of tissue from the brain of someone other than the patient or from an animal are required for long-lasting results. Our success in using a transplant of shark brain tissue into the brain of Parkinson's patients has been excellent. The shark tissue is well tolerated, and we look to this as medicine of the future.

Let us return to our thesis. Our first concern with the patient is to discover the cause of his disease. As we have previously discussed, we do not diagnose a symptom, but rather we search to find the deeper origin of the disease. If we learn that the patient suffered a skull injury many years ago, we recognize that this may be the cause of the present illness. In this case, we will give the patient hypothalamus cells. If he is very emotional, we will include limbic system, as well. In this case, to give lung tissue cells would not be wrong, but they would not be essential. If the patient has liver damage, liver tissue would be added. So, in this case, the patient would receive four different cells.

Do not mix the cells. They should be given separately, but in the same treatment and in the same day. Today's fine modern instruments can very accurately detect and prove scientifically if there are any symptoms of auto-immune activity (for example, ANA positive). In this event, you should be concerned about fiberblasts. One of the best sources of fiberblasts is in the umbilical cord. As we have noted, the embryo has no immune activity during the first three months, so the mother must send well-harmonized immune substances through the umbilical cord to protect the little embryo against any possible disease.

Multiple sclerosis is a prime example of an auto-immune disease that responds superbly to treatment. Before treatments, these patients will have a quotient of helper cells to suppresser cells of 20/1, which indicates over-activity of the helper cells, resulting in a disease such as MS. After treatment, the patient generally has a quotient of 2/1, which is approximately normal.

Parameters are crucially important and are to be considered much more seriously than the so-called "double-blind test," which has only created great confusion in modern medicine. The effects of the cell treatment involves weeks and, sometimes, even months. I reiterate that a high degree of moral and ethical responsibility should motivate the doctor and never the wish to simply charge large sums of money.

Excerpted from Professor Kühnau's Book, *Live-Cell Therapy: (Xenotransplants). My Life With a Medical Breakthrough.*

You can order his book through the product order form found in Appendix B.

Osteopathy

BY ARLEN L. BASS, D.O.

One may read in The World Book Encyclopedia, 1981

"OSTEOPATHY, or OSTEOPATHIC MEDICINE, is a system of medical practice that emphasizes the importance of the muscles and bones of the body and their connecting tendons, ligaments..."

And, I may add, that all-important fascia, the fibrous network that interconnects and envelops every structure, be it organ, blood vessel, nerve, bone or muscle, comprising the musculoskeletal system.

"Osteopathy maintains that the musculoskeletal system, which makes up sixty percent of the body, has important interrelationships with all other body systems. Osteopathy involves all aspects of medicine and includes various medical specialties. Osteopathic physicians use all the medical, surgical, immunological, pharmacological, psychological and hygienic procedures of modern medicine.

"Osteopathic physicians believe that a restriction or disturbance in the musculoskeletal system can lead to three main conditions. It can produce symptoms that occur only in the musculoskeletal system itself. It can cause symptoms resembling those of diseases that affect other body systems. And it can affect the functioning of other body systems connected to the musculoskeletal system through nerves and the action of hormones. Osteopathic physicians are specially trained in the detection and treatment of musculoskeletal disturbances."

To treat these, physical therapy is used, as well as massages and other types of active stretching, joint motion manipulation and passive osteopathic manipulation, such as fascial release, counterstrain by positioning, cranial and sacral guiding and balancing of hydraulic colloids in the fascial structures.

"This form of therapy is a distinctly osteopathic approach to the problems of health and disease."

My classmate Dr. Ed Stiles wrote about somatic dysfunction

"The musculoskeletal system makes up two-thirds of the total body mass and is a tremendous consumer of energy and materials while it performs its various functions. It is a major system that allows the host to respond to the stresses of life—physical, mental, emotional and spiritual. This puts a proportional demand on all tissues in the body to maintain the internal milieu. Somatic dysfunction can have an adverse effect on the sympathetic nervous system, which is the vasomotor system of the body, and thus can have a detrimental effect on arterial flow to all tissues of the body."

Nutritional aspects of fatigue

Because the gut and organs of digestion have to provide energy for the musculoskeletal as well as the other systems, the digestive system needs to function well. If one of the organisms that inhabit our intestines becomes dominant, then an imbalance in the chemicals of our internal environment will occur, like certain toxins produced by parasites or candida, whereas ideally many types of beneficial bacteria live symbiotically with us in our guts, as well as with each other: a diversity in harmony. As each uses the byproducts of the other, they may actually produce enzymes beneficial to our health. I'm beginning to believe that the colon should be more fertile than clean.

After my second year of osteopathic medical school, I worked as an orderly in an osteopathic hospital and learned about coffee enemas. I supposed it stimulated a tired colon. Into the colon of another patient who had had extensive antibiotic treatment, I received an order to instill a fecal enema. It made sense.

Fatigue

Psychic refers to the mind and nonphysical aspects of a person, and somatic refers to the physical body. Fatigue involves both. Hans Selye wrote about stress. Dr. Larry Jones wrote about strain. His concept of one muscle pulling on one side of a joint while its opposing muscle pulled on the other side of a joint has been very helpful to me and my patients. I tell them that these muscles are supposed to talk nicely to each other and take turns moving the joint in its particular direction. Jones's counterstrain is a way of teaching the muscles to communicate through the central nervous system and reach an agreement. It involves stretching the "bully" muscle and shortening the "victim" muscle just enough to quiet the latter's nerve control attachment, felt by the patient as a tender point under the physician's lightly palpating finger. Positioning the joint so that the point is not tender for ninety seconds constitutes a lesson session. Jones started teaching counterstrain in the early 1970s. I heard that it was more gentle than rolfing.

Freedom of motion

Another gentle manipulative treatment modality is the cranial and sacral concept researched initially by Dr. William G. Sutherland and taught to osteopaths in the 1940s. He realized in 1899 that the cranial bones were designed for motions and "respiratory" function "like the gills of a fish." At the time, he was a student at the first school of osteopathy in Kirksville, Missouri, founded by Dr. Andrew T. Still. He was inspired by Dr. Still's words that cerebrospinal fluid was the "highest known element" in the human body. Sutherland later learned the fluctuations of the cerebrospinal fluid and the rhythmic motions of the cranial bones and fascia, as well as the awful consequences of restriction of those motions. One of his experiments involved installing clamp screws to the leather football helmet that he put on to tighten down certain bones of his own head and restrict their motion. It wasn't just painful; it also affected his digestion and breathing. Once, he couldn't move his hands and had just enough strength left to call to his wife to come and unscrew the clamps.

Let's release the clamps

Thea is a sensitive and caring patient looking for answers to what has been called Chronic Fatigue Syndrome and Immune Dysfunction. She relates two severe traumatic blows to her head and pain where three bones connect together—the left parietal, occipital and mastoid portion of the temporal bone. The tissue memory is still palpable as motion restriction. This somatic dysfunction in the cranial area prevents full participation of the nerves in achieving homeostasis and health recovery. The brain lies in its waterbed of cerebrospinal fluid and relies on fluctuation of that fluid for nutrients. Tight occipital muscles jamming the head down on the first vertebra inhibit the proper functioning of the nerves to the neck muscles and is often found in what is being called depression. Releasing the compression of the vagus nerve helps the parasympathetic nervous system to better balance the sympathetic system, which, if irritable, inhibits peristalsis and digestion. Achieving freedom of the phrenic nerve by decompressing tight cranial bones and surrounding muscles allows relaxed diaphragmatic breathing. Patients may sigh or fall asleep on the treatment table. The pettipoint sign on the wall above the table says "It is more blessed to relieve." Thea feels head relief and tingling in her extremities.

What about fibromyalgia?

Chronic Fatigue Syndrome is probably more complex than toxins that accumulate in the muscles while they play tug of war. One of these byproducts of muscular activity is lactic acid, which acts as an irritant when it comes out of the muscle fibers and gets between them. It may be a vicious circle causing the muscle to tighten in defense, which in turn inhibits clearing the toxin by the blood and lymph fluids. This used to be called myofibrositis, a muscle fiber irritation, but now it has gained more notoriety with the algia suffix, meaning fiber and muscle pain. (Myofibralgia? No ring)

What about TMJ?

Thea tells me that a large percentage of chronic fatigue sufferers also have Temporomandibular Joint Syndrome, which is a complex membranous articular strain involving sensitive structures. The temporal bones contain the ears and connects with the occipital bone, through which the spinal cord passes, and with the sphenoid bone in the center of the head, which has a saddle where the pituitary gland sits, the reputed master of the endocrine system. Pretty important potentate!

Anyway, with strains of injuries or even prolonged uterine contractions on the infant's skull during birth, patterns are established that can be asymmetrical. This is called plagiocephaly, meaning twisted head. I cringed while watching a TV program a few years back about a little girl who underwent extensive skull surgery to "correct" a misshapen head, which most probably would have responded to a series of gentle molding manipulative treatments from a cranial osteopath.

The temporal bones can be less severely held in an asymmetrical strain pattern, which will result in one TMJ being more forward than the other and causing the jaw to shift more to the other side. One of the muscles controlling it attaches to the cartilage cushion between the jaw and the fossa in the temporal bone, and if that pterygoid muscle gets into a strain habit, it pulls the cushion out of place when chewing, perhaps resulting in painful popping. One must achieve proper symmetry of the bones and balance between opposing muscles. Oral myofunctional therapists can help by retraining mouth muscle habits, but they are as scarce as cranial osteopaths.

Why aren't all osteopaths trained in craniosacral therapy?

As you can read in encyclopedias, osteopathic physicians are fully trained in the medical tradition, and most want to provide their services as general family primary-care doctors. In order to pay off their medical school loans, some will serve as emergency room physicians, enter residencies for specialty training or otherwise become caught up in the medical doctor mold. They may not have had time to sit down and let their hands listen to the body and head tissues. Because of this, another of my classmates, John Upledger, D.O., began teaching the craniosacral concept to massage therapists and others who are good with their hands. There is a need for anatomical treatment that few yet know they have. Thank you, Thea Schlosser, for your concern that people get the help that they need.

This I Know

By Bari Maddock, D. MSc.

...that the miracle of birth gave me an opportunity to experience this life, this planet, these challenges, these myriad adventures, involvements, and ordeals in order that I may gain understanding and wisdom.

...that I am a unique, original, and wonderful being. There is not another human on this earth like me. This means that I am unequaled. Everything about me is individual from my fingerprints to my smile, my walk to my thought.

...that I have the freedom to express anything I choose through this body that I occupy. This is the greatest gift possible.

...that I am the master of my life. Despite my obstacles, handicaps, traumas, I AM. There is no human power on this earth capable of controlling my thoughts unless I give them that power.

...that health is composed of three things: attitude, diet, and exercise, and the greatest of these is attitude. Without a belief in self, a knowingness of self-worth, a love of self, the body is blocked from realizing the full value of the other two.

...that if I do not learn from experience, life will present it again and again with infinite patience until I have finally achieved wisdom and can move on to new and exciting challenges.

...that I cannot own another person nor can I make another responsible for my happiness. Only I have that power and if I give it to another, only I will reap the bitter fruits of disappointment.

...that when I point a finger at another, the three that are pointing at me magnify three-fold in myself the virtues or vices I am emphasizing in the other.

...that yesterday and all the yesterdays before are gone and tomorrow is still a nebulous possibility. But I have this glorious day—this now, this moment—that will never come again. I have the gift of this newness complete and whole to do with as I choose.

...These things I know—for me. It is my fervent desire that you also know them for you.

Bari Maddock is a holistic psychologist. Her undergraduate work was done at UCLA, and she completed a doctorate at California Coast University and the University of Metaphysics in Los Angeles, CA. Extensive studies in nutrition, esoteric science, yoga, creative imagery, and modification have all contributed to her threefold approach to well-being. Dr. Maddock has recovered from CFS and personal tragedies to be a living testament to her teachings.

The Possible Connection of Prions and CFIDS

By Professor Wolfram Kühnau, M.D.

During the recent past there has been much discussion in the international press about the so-called "mad cow" disease and an obvious relation to the extremely dangerous Creuzfeldt-Jakob Disease. Material from dried brain cells of cows that had died of this disease were injected into rats and other laboratory animals, showing clearly that the disease can be transmitted to other animals. It is to the great credit of Dr. Prusiner, University of California Medical School, San Francisco, that it was found that the contagious agent was a so-called "prion," a protein that has no DNA and RNA and cannot be killed with cooking or usual disinfectants.

So, we are confronted with an absolutely new situation and a "third form" of life that was, until now, unknown. We have known of three prions until now; it can be supposed that many more of them can be detected, even those that are much less aggressive and less dangerous. It has been proven that the first animals having a dangerous prion is the sheep. Since the English and Zealanders are using deposits of sheep as fertilizers in the fields, this is a way of spreading out the prion.The pigs then eat the herbs that are growing in these fields, and then, finally, the cows graze in these fields and get sick and die.

There are reports now that the so-called "Desert Storm" disease is practically identical with CFIDS and some investigators have found a lot of dead sheep in the Desert War. It is possible that a prion could be the agent that is causing the Chronic Fatigue and Immune Disorder Syndrome. It makes sense that those patients have normal or practically normal blood tests and that all the classical clinical trials are normal because, with the absence of RNA and DNA, the human body has no possibility to develop antibodies, etc. As we also know now, the AIDS virus cannot work without a former action of a prion *(New York Times,* May 10, 1996), so we must seriously investigate the possibility that the true cause of CFIDS is a prion.

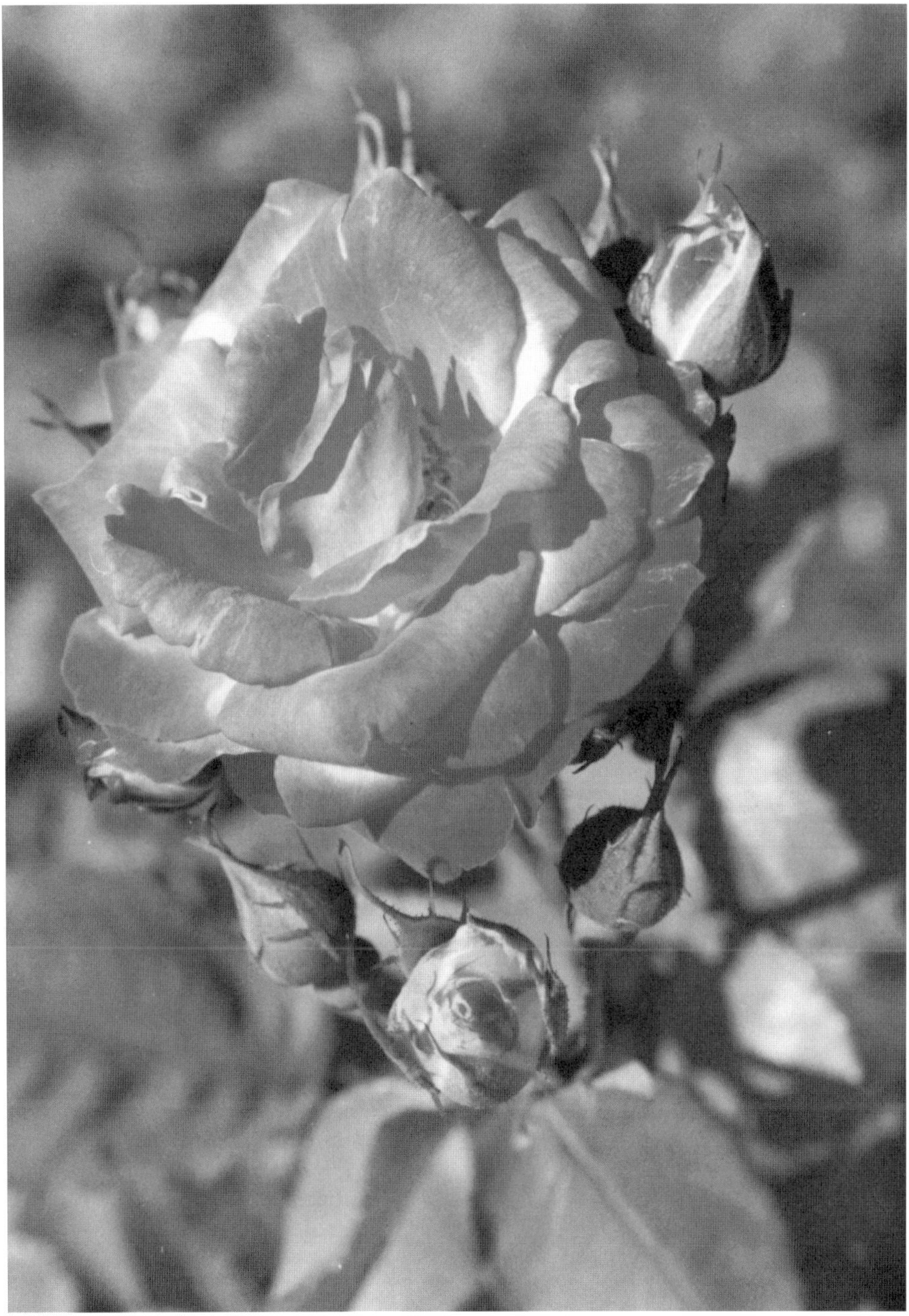

Photo by Thea.

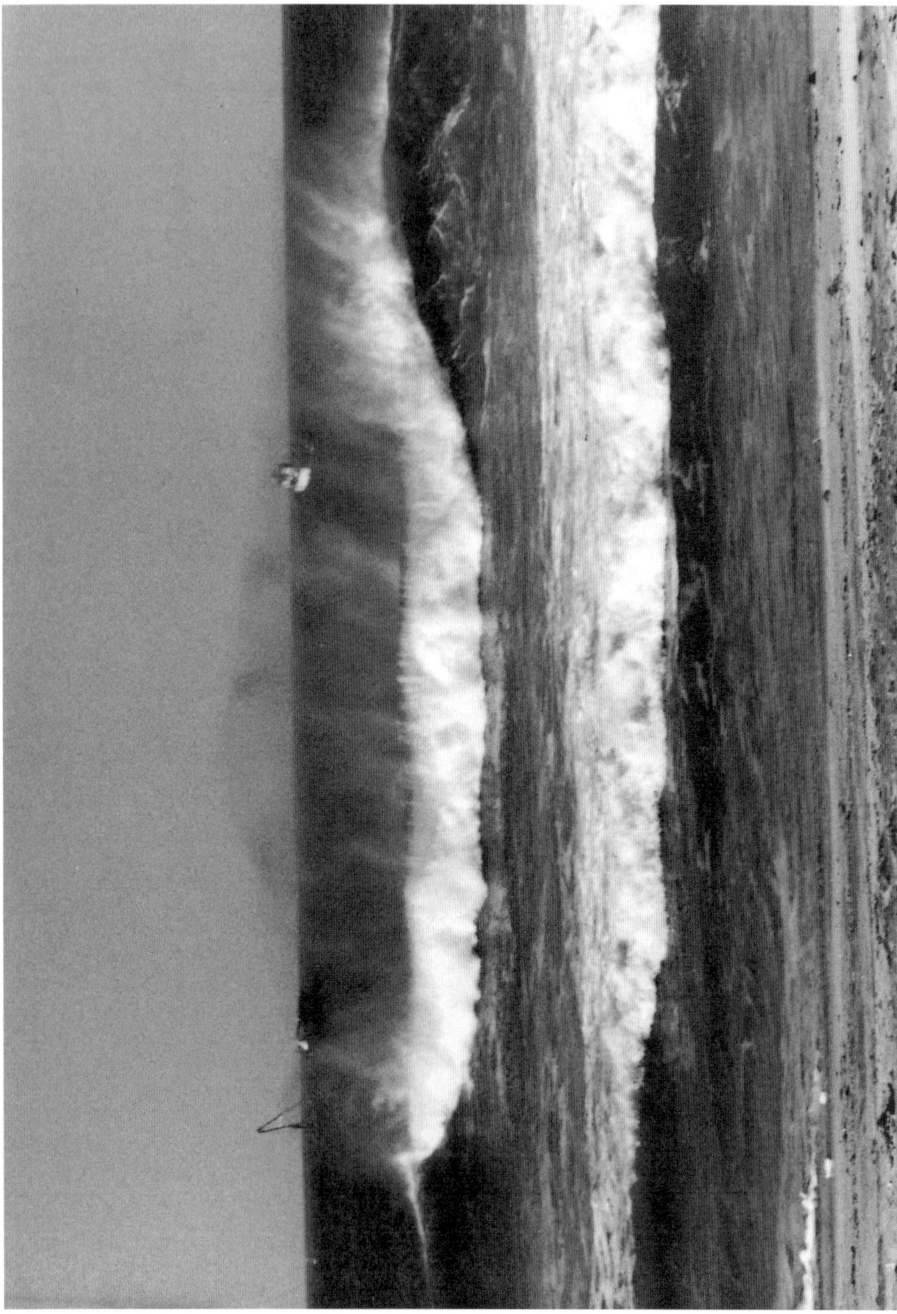

Photo by Thea. Rosarita Beach, Mexico, 1989.

Appendix B

- CFS Symptom Checklist
- Chronic Fatigue and Immune Dysfunction Media Awareness Association
- CFIDS Buyer's Club
- The National CFS Foundation
- The CFIDS Association of America Inc.
- The CFIDS Foundation
- Kayser's Nutrition Centers
- L.M. Caldwell Pharmacist
- Efficient Systems, President Steven Boehm
- Your Product Order List
- Selected Bibliography
- Epilogue

Dr. Jay A. Goldstein M.D.
The CFS Institute
6200 E. Canton Rim Road #110-D
Anaheim Hills, CA 92807
(714) 998-2780

CFS Symptom Checklist

This symptom checklist is not sufficient to diagnose Chronic Fatigue Syndrome unless other disorders have been ruled out by appropriate assessment.

A. Did your illness begin: ☐ abruptly ☐ gradually
at age?____ age now____?

B. Did your illness begin with a flu-like episode? ☐ yes ☐ no
If yes: were lab tests done?__________
What tests?____

____

Were abnormalities found?________________________________

C. Were you treated for psychological problems prior to the onset of this illness? ☐ yes ☐ no
If yes: psychotherapy? ☐ yes ☐ no

Medication:____

D. Did your illness follow exposure to new carpet/paint, tung oil, industrial solvents, pesticides, or other environmental toxins?
☐ yes ☐ no
If yes, please describe:__________________________________

E. Were you subjected to prolonged stressors during childhood (e.g., abusive or dysfunctional home)? ☐ yes ☐ no

If yes, please describe:________________________________

F. Were you subjected to unusual or extreme stressors in your life immediately prior to the onset of this illness? ☐ yes ☐ no

If yes, please describe:________________________________

G. Have you had silicone breast implants? ☐ yes ☐ no

Have you had silicone injections? ☐ yes ☐ no

Have you had collagen injections? ☐ yes ☐ no

If yes to any of the above, did you have these procedures before or after the onset of your CFS symptoms? ☐ before ☐ after

H. Are your symptoms worse: ☐ in the summer ☐ in the winter

☐ no difference

RATE THE SEVERITY OF YOUR SYMPTOMS FROM 0 TO 10:

1. _____Fatigue, usually made worse by physical exercise

Is your level of activity less than 50% of normal?

☐ yes ☐ no

2. _____Cognitive function problems

____ a) attention deficit disorder, including concentration problems

____ b) calculation difficulties

(describe) ________________________________

____

____ c) memory disturbance

(describe) ________________________________

____

____ d) spatial disorientation, getting lost in familiar locations, problems judging distances

____ e) frequently saying the wrong word

3. _____Psychological problems

____ a) depression

____ b) anxiety, which may include panic attacks and phobias

___ c) personality changes, usually worsening of a previous mild tendency

___ d) emotional ability (mood swings)

___ e) psychosis

4. ____ Other nervous system problems

___ a) sleep disturbance

___ b) headaches

___ c) changes in visual activity

___ d) seizures

___ e) numb or tingling feelings

___ f) light-headedness, feeling "spaced out"

___ g) disequilibrium

___ h) frequent unusual nightmares

___ i) difficulty moving your tongue to speak

___ j) ringing in ears

___ k) paralysis

___ l) severe muscular weakness

___ m) blackouts

___ n) intolerance of bright lights

___ o) intolerance of alcohol

___ p) alteration of taste, smell and hearing

___ q) non-restorative sleep

___ r) decreased libido

___ s) twitching muscles (benign fasciculation)

5. ____Recurrent flu-like illnesses, often with chronic sore throat

6. ____Painful lymph nodes, especially in nodes of neck and under the arms

7. ____Several nasal and other allergies, often worsening of previous mild problem

8. ____Weight change, usually a gain
9. ____Muscle and joint aches with tender "trigger points" or fibromyalgia
10. ___Abdominal pain, diarrhea, nausea, intestinal gas, "irritable bowel syndrome"
11. ___ Low-grade fevers or feeling hot often
12 ___ Night sweats
13. ___Heart palpitations
14. ___Severe premenstrual syndrome, PMS
15. ___Rash of Herpes simplex or shingles
16. ___Uncomfortable or recurrent urination, pain in prostate
17. ___Other symptoms:
    ___ a) rashes
    ___ b) hair loss
    ___ c) impotence
    ___ d) chest pain
    ___ e) dry eyes and mouth
    ___ f) cough
    ___ g) TMJ syndrome
    ___ h) endometriosis
    ___ i) frequent canker sores
    ___ j) cold hands and feet
    ___ k) serious rhythm disturbances of the heart
    ___ l) carpal tunnel syndrome
    ___ m) pyriform muscle syndrome causing sciatica
    ___ n) thyroid inflammation
    ___ o) various cancers
    ___ p) periodontal (gum) disease
    ___ q) mitral valve prolapse

___ r) easily getting out of breath (“dyspnea on exertion”)
___ s) symptoms worsened by extremes of temperature
___ t) multiple sensitivities to medicine, food, and other substances

Chronic Fatigue and Immune Dysfunction Media Awareness Association

Founder Thea Schlosser

Chronic Fatigue and Immune Dysfunction
Media Awareness Association
P.O. Box 41028, Santa Barbara, California 93140
Fax: (805) 969-7669 • Phone or Fax: (805) 963-7799

Beyond The Dark Cloud may also be purchased at the above address for $19.95 (outside USA $22.45). Please include $4.50 for shipping and handling, plus California sales tax of 7.75%. Include $6.00 for priority mail. Please add $11.00 for orders outside the USA.

All photographs in this book are available in 11x14 color enlargements (two in black and white only), signed by Thea, for $85.00.

The Chronic Fatigue and Immune Dysfunction Media Awareness Association is dedicated to increasing the awareness of CFIDS. We would like to hear from you. Please write us with personal accounts, poems, suggestions, tips, or whatever else you may want to share.

Donations for Chronic Fatigue and Immune Dysfunction research and more media coverage would be very much appreciated.

We are working on a quarterly newsletter that would include up-to-date information on CFIDS. We will begin distribution in September of 1996. A yearly subscription will be $30.00.

Thank you so much,

Thea

You may also find the following sources useful in obtaining information about CFIDS.

CFIDS Buyer's Club

Founded by Rich Carson, the CFIDS Buyer's Club is one of the largest fund-raisers for CFIDS research raising 1.8 million dollars to date! They offer more than 120 high-quality nutritional supplements. They also publish Healthwatch, a quarterly newsletter containing invaluable, up-to-date information, as well as the latest research on CFIDS. 1-800-366-6056. Call today for your FREE catalogue.

The National CFS Foundation

3521 Broadway, Suite 222, Kansas City, MO 64111

The CFIDS Association of America Inc.

PO Box 220398, Charlotte, NC 28222-0398
1-800-44-CFIDS (23437)

The CFIDS Foundation

965 Mission Street, San Francisco, CA 94103

The Nightingale Research Foundation

383 Danforth Avenue, Ottawa, Ontario, Canada K2A OE3

Kayser's Nutrition Centers

1-800-242-FLIP, ask for Steve

L.M. Caldwell Pharmacist

Will deliver or mail prescriptions if you are unable to leave your home.
235 W. Pueblo Street, Santa Barbara, CA 93105
(805) 682-7353

Arlen L. Bass, O.D.

1200 De la Vina Street, Santa Barbara, CA 93101
(805) 966-9914

Efficient Systems, Steven Boehm

665 Coyote Road, Santa Barbara, CA 93108
(805) 969-4948

YOUR PRODUCT ORDER LIST

Please send check or money order to:
CFIDS Media Awareness Association
P.O. Box 41028, Santa Barbara, California 93140
Fax (805) 969-7669 • Phone or Fax (805) 963-7799

NAME OF PRODUCT		QTY	PRICE EACH	TOTAL
Beyond The Dark Cloud	USA Outside Country		$19.95 $23.00	
"Xenotransplant Therapy," a book by Professor Wolfram Kühnau, M.D. English or Spanish			$18.00	
Thea's videotape interview of Dr. Kühnau treating illness with Xenotransplants Audio tape only			$24.95 $12.50	
Videotape by Dr. Jay Goldstein and Thea Schlosser on CFIDS "Growing Younger," with host Elisa Henley Frerra Audio tape only			$24.95 $12.50	
CFIDS Media Awareness Association Quarterly Newsletter beginning Sept. 96			Year $30.00	
Videotape on CFIDS, Cancer, AIDS and Xenotransplant Therapy, Professor Wolfram Kühnau, M.D. and Thea Schlosser, with host Elvera Boile, "Past, Present and Future" Audio tape only			$24.95 $12.50	
Each color photograph in the book (two in black & white only), enlarged to 11x14 and signed by Thea			$85.00	
Life Guard—Advanced Anti-Oxidant Therapy *I've researched many antioxidants and have found Life Guard to be one of the best —Thea*			60 Tablets $38.50	

Name (please print) ______________________

Street Address ______________________

City/State/Zip ______________________

Please indicate payment method:

☐ **Check or Money Order Enclosed for $** ______________

☐ **Visa** ☐ **MasterCard Card No.** ______________

Exp. Date __________ **Signature** ______________

Subtotal	
CA Tax (7.75%)	
Shipping & Handling Priority Mail Outside country	$ 4.50 $ 6.00 $11.00
Total	

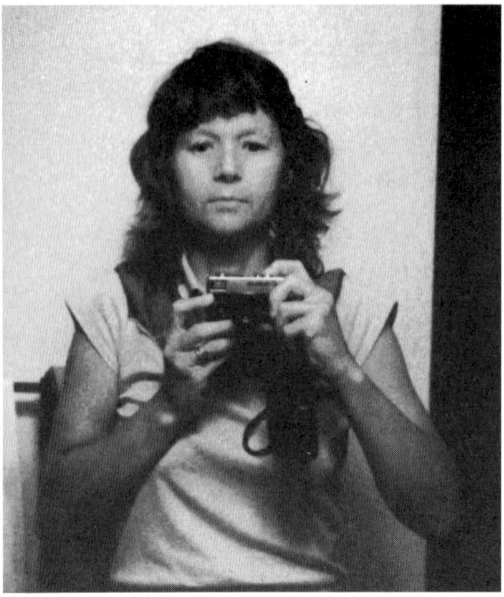 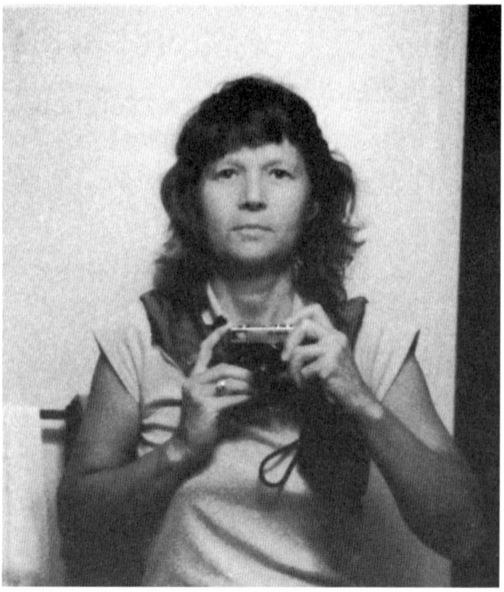

These pictures were taken in 1983. I told my doctor that I felt ill and exhausted. I had severe edema (water retention) throughout my body. He told me that I was OK and sent me home—I went to see someone else. Shortly after that, they performed a thyroid panel on me. We were shocked at the results. The measurement for my T4 was only 1.5. A normal reading is between 4.5 and 13! It took three months to get me on my feet again. I put these photos in the back of the book as one last reminder to all physicians. Please listen to your patients closely before saying that there is nothing wrong.

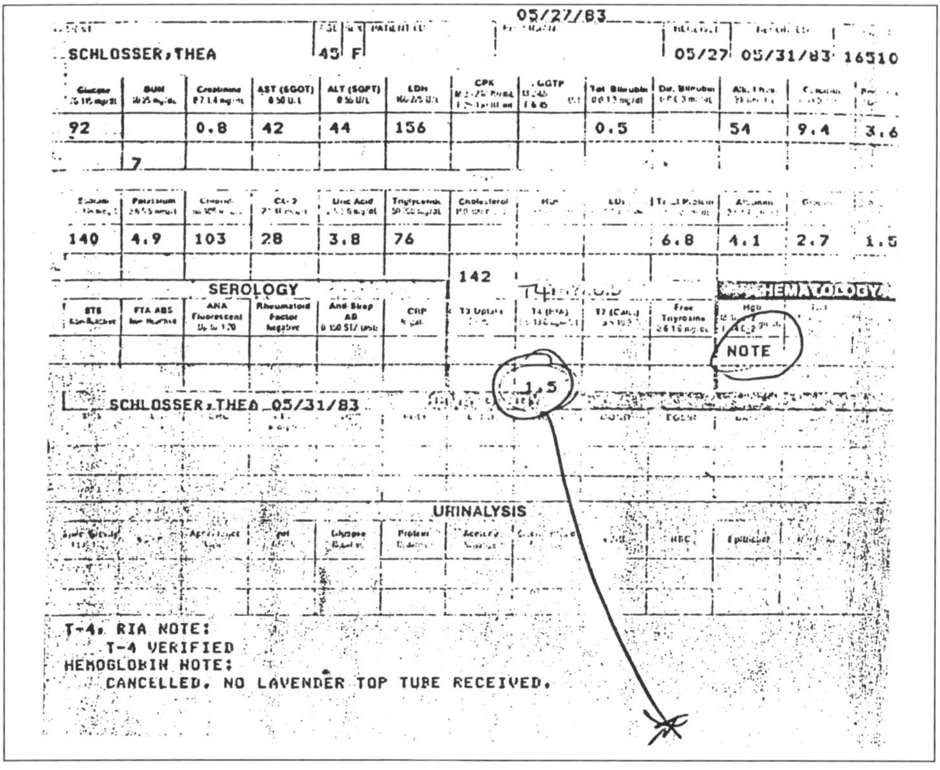

05/27/83

SCHLOSSER, THEA 43 F 05/27 05/31/83 16510

Glucose	BUN	Creatinine	AST (SGOT)	ALT (SGPT)	LDH	CPK	GGTP	Tot. Bilirubin	Dir. Bilirubin	Alk. Phos.	Calcium	
92		0.8	42	44	156			0.5		54	9.4	3.6
	7											

Sodium	Potassium	Chloride	CO2	Uric Acid	Triglycerides	Cholesterol	HDL	LDL	Total Protein	Albumin	Globulin	
140	4.9	103	28	3.8	76				6.8	4.1	2.7	1.5
						142						

SEROLOGY

STS	FTA ABS	ANA Fluorescent	Rheumatoid Factor	Anti-Strep AB	CRP	T3 Uptake	T4 (RIA)	T7 (Calc.)	Free Thyroxine
							1.5		

HEMATOLOGY

Hgb

NOTE

SCHLOSSER, THEA 05/31/83

URINALYSIS

T-4, RIA NOTE:
T-4 VERIFIED
HEMOGLOBIN NOTE:
CANCELLED. NO LAVENDER TOP TUBE RECEIVED.

Selected Bibliography

Ali, M.D., Majid "The Canary of Chronic Fatigue."

Balch, M.D., James *Prescription for Nutritional Healing.*

Berne, Ph.D., Katrina H. "CFIDS Lite."

Berne, Ph.D., Katrina H. "Running On Empty."

Black, M.D., Arthur P. "A New Diagnostic Method in Allergic Disease." Pediatrics, May 1956, pp. 171-176.

Braly, M.D., James "Food Allergy and Nutrition Revolution."

Crook, M.D., William G. "Chronic Fatigue and the Yeast Connection."

Culbert, DsC., Michael "AIDS: Hope, Hoax and Hoopla."

Culbert, DsC., Michael "CFS—Conquering the Crippler."

Digest of Alternative Medicine, 1-800-683-7014.

Feiden, Karyn "Hope and Help For CFIDS."

Fisher, G. "Chronic Fatigue Syndrome: A Victim's Guide."

Forman, Ph.D., Robert "How to Control Your Allergies." New York: Larchmont Books, 1979.

Fry, J. "Infectious Mononucleosis, Some New Observations From a 15 Year Study." Fam. Pract. 1980, 10:1087.

Goldstein, M.D., Jay A. "Chronic Fatigue Syndrome: The Limbic Hypothesis."

Goldstein, M.D., Jay A. "Portrayal of the Brain."

Gordon, M.D., Jay *Good Foods Today—Great Kids Tomorrow.*

Gregory, O.M.D., Scott J. "A Holistic Protocol for Immune System."

Holmes, G.P., Kaplan, J.E., Gantz, N.M., Komaroff, A.L., et al. Chronic Fatigue Syndrome: A working case definition. *Annals of Internal Medicine* 108:387-389, 1988.

Hyde, M.D., Byron Marshall "The Clinical and Scientific Basis of Myalgic Encephalomyelitis Chronic Fatigue Syndrome." (From the Nightingale Research Foundation.)

Kaslow, M.D., Arthur L. "Freedom From Chronic Disease." Los Angeles: J.P. Tarcher, Inc. 1979.

Konlee, Mark "How to Reverse Immune Dysfunction."

Kugler, Ph.D., Hans "Tripping the Clock."

Kühnau, M.D., Professor Wolfram "Live-Cell Therapy (Xenotransplants)."

Mendelson, M.D., Robert "Confessions of a Medical Heretic." N.Y.: Warner Books.

Mowrey, Ph.D., Daniel *Herbal Tonic Therapies.*

Nicolson, G.L. and Nicolson, N.L. Chronic Fatigue Illness and Operation Desert Storm. *Journal of Occupational and Environmental Medicine* 38:14-16, 1996.

Ostram, Neeya "50 Things You Should Know About the Chronic Fatigue Syndrome Epidemic."

Passwater, Richard A. "Supernutrition Megavitamin Revolution." N.Y. Pocketbooks, 1979.

Rosenbaum, M.D., M. and Susser, M.D., M. "Solving the Puzzle of Chronic Fatigue Syndrome."

Schmidt, P., Blanck, R.M. Gulf War Syndrome and CFS. *CFIDS Chronicle* 8: 25-27, 1995.

Shepherd, Dr. Charles "Living With M.E."

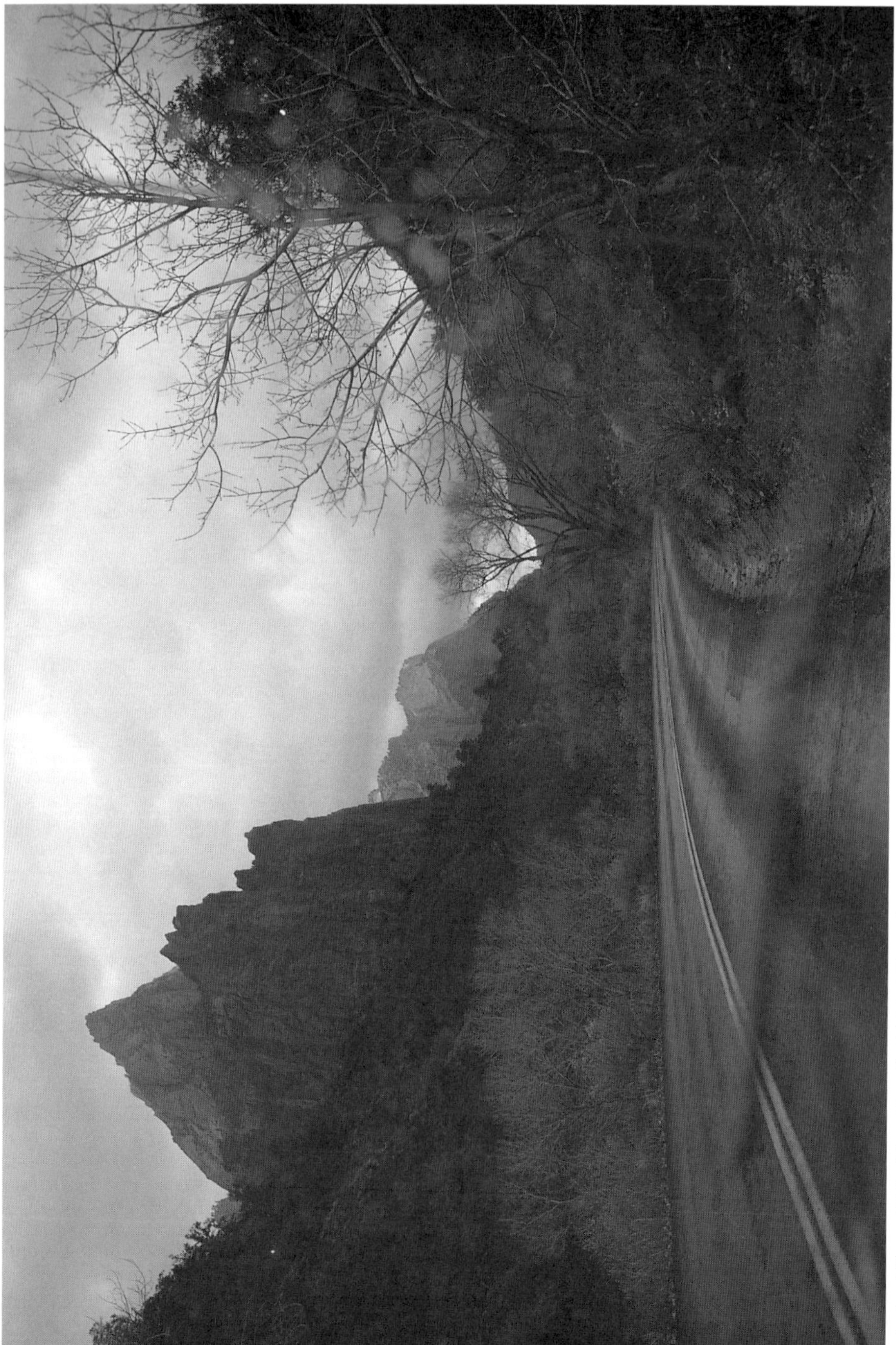

Photo by Thea. Winding Road, 1982, Zion Canyon.

Epilogue

The preceding pages and chapters have provided an overview of Chronic Fatigue and Immune Dysfunction Syndrome. As previously stated, science has only begun to unlock the mysterious symptoms surrounding CFIDS.

More research will eventually give us a better understanding and hopefully a cure. There is also much research being done on AIDS, which in turn will help CFIDS, since both are diseases of the immune system.

Worldwide, researchers are working on solving immune dysfunction diseases.

I have shared with all of you my personal experiences, some of which were very difficult to put down on paper. But this is one of the responsibilities that come with the undertaking of a project such as this one.

Just when I thought *Beyond The Dark Cloud* was totally finished, I decided to look for a photograph that might give added meaning to the end of the book. With eagerness and hope, I looked through my photography collection. Sure enough, I found just what I was looking for with the photograph called *Winding Road,* 1982, Zion Canyon.

As I mentioned in the book previously, recovering from CFIDS feels like reaching the top of the highest mountain on a winding, and, at times, invisible road. As difficult as it might feel—that *recovery is impossible*—I feel ***recovery is possible.***

Until then, let there be hope and healing.

—Thea

Personal Notes